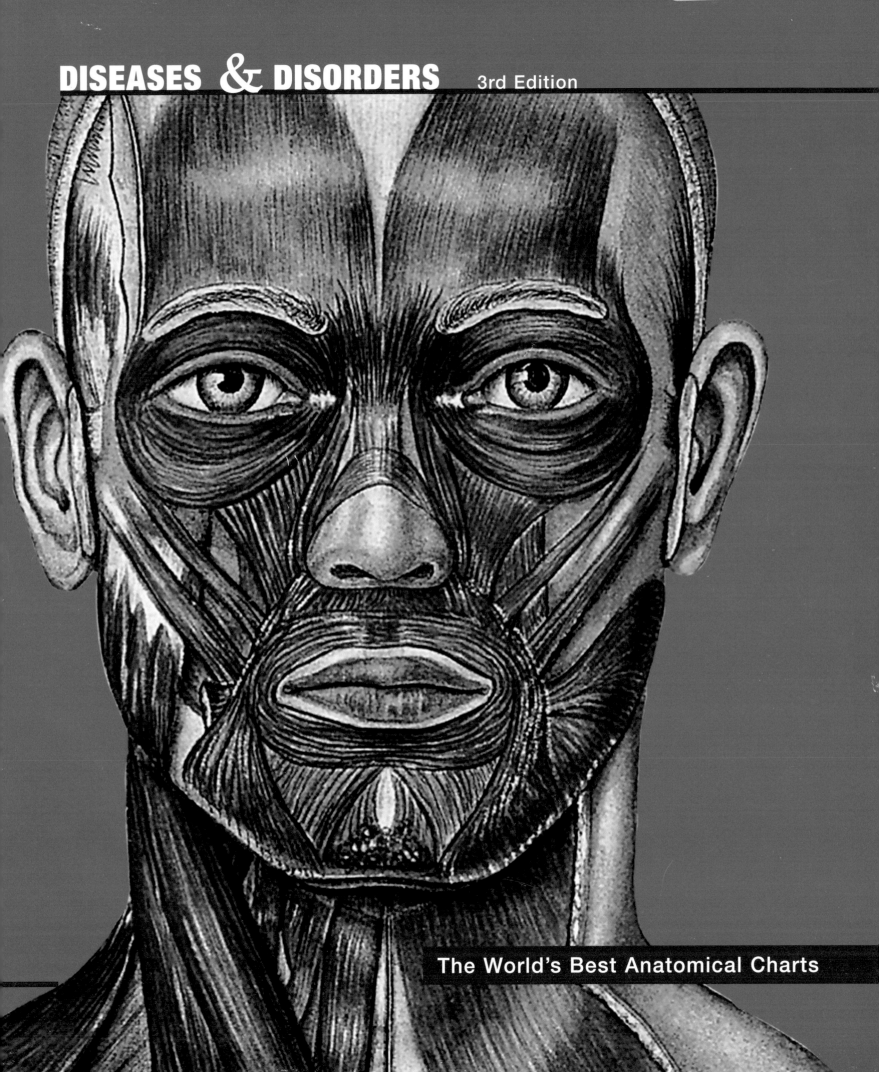

DISEASES & DISORDERS 3rd Edition

The World's Best Anatomical Charts

CONTENTS

Copyright ©2000, 2005, 2008 Wolters Kluwer Health Lippincott Williams & Wilkins

Published by **Anatomical Chart Company, Skokie, IL USA**

3rd Edition
ISBN 10: 0-7817-8211-2
ISBN 13: 978-0-7817-8211-1   Library of Congress Control Number: 2007932843

Understanding Depression

What Is Depression?

Depression is a serious medical condition that affects thoughts, moods, feelings, behavior, and physical health. There are different types of depressions, the most common is Major Depressive Disorder. Major Depressive Disorder and other types of serious depressions are "long-lasting" and get in the way of a person's ability to work, study, sleep, and eat.

Signs and Symptoms of Major Depression

A person may have depression if five or more of the following symptoms are present for more than two weeks at any one time; this should be reported to a healthcare provider.

- Loss of interest or enjoyment in normal daily activities
- Persistent sad, anxious, or hopeless mood
- Irritability or nervousness
- Feelings of guilt, fear, or worthlessness
- Significant weight loss or gain due to appetite change
- Overtiredness and/or decreased energy
- Unable to sleep or too much sleep
- Unexplained crying spells
- Difficulty concentrating, remembering, and/or making decisions
- Little or no interest in companionship or sex
- Thoughts of death or suicide

If thoughts of suicide exist, or if symptoms get in the way of daily activities, one should seek treatment right away.

Who is at Risk for Depression?

Although depression can be triggered by personal problems, other factors also affect who becomes depressed. Often, a combination of risk factors are involved.

- **Heredity:** Some types of depression run in families. However, not everyone with a family history of depression will develop the disorder.
- **Gender:** Twice as many women as men experience depression.
- **Hormonal Changes:** Changing hormone levels, as in the post-partum period, may cause depression.
- **Alcohol and Drug Abuse**
- **Medications:** Certain drugs can cause depression, so it is important for patients to provide a complete list of medications to their health care provider.
- **Physical Disease:** Illnesses such as stroke, heart attack, cancer, Parkinson's disease, hormonal disorders and viral infections can cause depression.
- **Stress:** Traumatic experiences, such as the loss of a love one, can trigger depression.

Areas of the Brain Affected by Depression

Some areas of the brain are underactive in depression, while other areas are over- active. These changes contribute to the emotional and physical symptoms of depression

Thalamus
Controls a person's degree of arousal and awareness, including sleep and hypervigilance. It stimulates the amygdala. The thalamus is highly active in people with depression.

Hypothalamus
Produces the neurotransmitters that are involved in mood and emotional expressions. Serotonin pathways in the hypothalamus help regulate mood and appetite while norepinephrine pathways help regulate emotions and energy level.

Amygdala
Responsible for negative feelings; it is highly active in people with depression.

Anterior cingulate cortex
Helps associate smells and sights with pleasant memories. It also has a role in emotional response to pain and the regulation of anger. This area is highly active in people with depression.

Prefrontal cortex
Involved in complex thinking, personality, and social behavior. Norepinephrine and serotonin are two neurotransmitters that affect mood in this part of the brain. Norepinephrine pathways impact attention span, concentration, memory, and information processing. There is decreased activity in the prefrontal cortex in depression.

The Limbic System

Regulates emotions, instincts, motivations and sexual drive. It also plays a role in the body's response to stress. Any disturbances to the limbic system can affect mood and behavior.

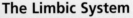

Hippocampus

Amygdala

Fornix

Thalamus

Mamillary body

The Role of Neurotransmitters

Neurotransmitters are chemicals that carry messages between the nerve cells (neurons); these affect behavior, mood, and thought. Depression is related to these chemical imbalances in the brain.

Abnormal

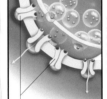

With low levels of norepinephrine and serotonin neurotransmitters, membrane channels do not open; as a result, nerve messages are not passed on, and areas of the brain that affect emotions may not receive stimulation. This process may result in depression.

Closed membrane channels seen on a neuron affected by depression

Normal

Opened membrane channels seen on a neuron not affected by depression

Other Types of Depression

Dysthymic Disorder (Dysthymia)

Dysthymic disorder is a milder, more chronic form of depression compared to major depressive disorder. A person may feel depressed one day and normal on another day. Although the symptoms are not as disabling, having dysthymia increases the risk of developing major depression.

Bipolar Disorder (Manic-Depressive Illness)

Bipolar disorder is described as recurring cycles of intense moods. A person may experience recurrent "high" moods (mania), very "low" moods (depression), or switching between these highs and lows. During the "highs", one may be too confident, very talkative, energetic, impulsive and take high risks. One may also get very little sleep, be very irritable, and make poor decisions. During the "lows", one may appear depressed and unable to concentrate.

Suicide

People who are depressed are at higher risk for suicide. If a person feels life is not worth living, especially if one is thinking about ending his/her life, seek treatment immediately.
Any threat of suicide should be taken seriously. Contact a mental health professional or suicide hotline immediately if you experience any of the following danger signs.

- Pacing, nervous behavior, frequent mood changes (this symptom by itself is not an emergency or suggestive of being suicidal)
- Actions or threats of physical harm or violence
- Threats or talking of death or suicide
- Withdrawal from activities and relationships (by itself, this is not an emergency)
- Giving away prized possessions or saying goodbye to friends
- A sudden brightening of mood after a period of severe depression
- Unusually risky behavior

Treatment

Depression can almost always be treated effectively. Certain medications and medical conditions can also cause the same symptoms as depression; the diagnosis of depression must be made by a health professional. If depression is diagnosed, treatment can include one or more of the following:

Antidepressants

These medications rebalance key chemicals, neurotransmitters, in the brain and take time to work. Neurotransmitters are required for the brain to function normally. A variety of antidepressants may be tried before finding the treatment that may work best for you.

Counseling (Psychotherapy)

Counseling involves talking with a trained mental health professional. It helps people gain insight into their feelings and learn how to deal with them, change behaviors, and resolve problems.

Mood Stabilizers

These medications help soothe mood swings. Many people with bipolar disorder may take mood stabilizers to "even out" their moods.

Alternative Therapies

- **Herbal therapy** may have a beneficial effect on mild cases of depression. Talk to your healthcare provider before taking any herbal or dietary supplement.
- **Regular Exercise** can ease the symptoms of mild depression. Research indicates that physical activity has a positive effect on brain chemicals, which can improve mood and sense of well being.

Understanding Epilepsy

What Is Epilepsy?

Epilepsy is a common neurological condition that affects millions of people throughout the world. The term "epilepsy" is a general name that refers to many different disorders in which people tend to experience seizures. Other conditions, such as high fever, the use of or withdrawal from drugs or alcohol, or a blow to the head, can cause an isolated seizure. Only those people who have had two or more seizures are diagnosed as having epilepsy.

What Causes Epilepsy?

Many cases of epilepsy are said to be symptomatic. This means they are the result of other conditions such as a birth injury, head injury, stroke, brain tumor, infection, or congenital abnormality. Genetic factors may also play a role in the cause of epilepsy. Some cases of epilepsy, however, remain idiopathic, meaning they develop for reasons which we presently cannot determine.

How the Brain Works

Although it appears to be solid, the brain is made up of billions of cells, including a network of cells called neurons. These neurons branch out, much like branches on a tree. This neural network enables communication within the brain and between the brain and the rest of the body.

Neurons

When a neuron "fires" it sends small electrical impulses along its branches toward surrounding cells. At the end of each branch is a small gap or synapse, which the impulse must overcome in order to continue its journey.

When an impulse reaches the end of a branch, chemicals called neurotransmitters are released to flood the synapse. Some are excitatory, stimulating the neighboring cell to fire. Others are inhibitory, making the next cell less likely to fire.

The brain's ability to turn electrical impulses "on" and "off" allows it to control messages and work effectively. Since normal behavior is the result of many neurons working together, a fine balance of excitatory and inhibitory factors is needed to insure that the correct neurons fire at the appropriate times. In people with epilepsy, however, this fine balance is upset, making the brain unable to limit the spread of electrical activity. When too many neurons fire at once, an electrical storm is created within the brain.

Vesicles release neurotransmitters, which flood the synapse.

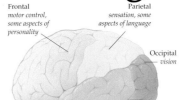

Frontal
motor control, some aspects of personality

Parietal
sensation, some aspects of language

Occipital
vision

Temporal
speech, hearing

The brain is divided into two hemispheres. The right half controls the left side of the body and the left half controls the right side of the body. Each hemisphere is divided into four lobes. Within the lobes there are even smaller areas, each associated with specific functions.

What Is a Seizure?

A seizure is an excessive discharge of electrical activity within the brain, which leads to a change in movement, sensation, experience, or consciousness. There are many types of seizures. The effects they have on the body vary greatly, depending on where in the brain the seizure starts and where it spreads.

Seizures Can Cause:

- A twitching muscle
- Convulsive movements
- A tingling sensation
- Sweating
- The perception of an unusual smell or taste
- Hallucinations
- Fear or anxiety
- Changes in awareness
- Loss of consciousness
- Other changes

This illustration shows a seizure originating in the left motor strip, affecting movement of the fingers, hand, and arm.

Phases of a Seizure

Aura: an unusual sensation or peculiar feeling often felt prior to a more widespread seizure. Can also be called a simple partial seizure.

Ictus: the whole seizure, including the aura.

Post-ictus: time after a seizure; may experience muscle weakness or deep sleep.

If Someone Has a Seizure

Although big seizures may be frightening to witness, they are usually not medical emergencies. In most cases the seizure itself is not harmful to the individual who is having it and therefore should be allowed to run its course. An ambulance is usually not necessary unless the seizure lasts longer than five minutes, there are multiple, repeated seizures, or the person is injured, diabetic or pregnant. There is nothing family or friends can do to stop a seizure, but certain steps can be taken to prevent further injury.

You Should:

- Stay calm
- Help the person lie down and roll onto one side to prevent choking
- Loosen tight, restrictive clothing and remove eyeglasses
- Protect the person's head with a soft object such as a pillow or jacket
- Gently guide a conscious but confused person away from hazards
- Remain with the person until she/he is awake and alert
- Be comforting and reassuring

You Should Not:

- Put anything into the person's mouth
- Try to restrain the person

Generalized Seizures

These seizures affect both hemispheres of the brain at the same time. Abnormal activity is not focused in one specific area and there generally is no aura at the start.

Main Forms of Generalized Seizures

- **Typical absence seizures** (formerly called "petit mal") – result in brief episodes of impaired awareness. There also may be small motor movements, changes in muscle tone, or automatic behaviors.
- **Atonic seizures** – associated with a sudden loss of muscle tone in a limb or throughout the entire body. The person having the seizure will often drop things or fall to the ground.
- **Myoclonic seizures** – sudden shock-like jolt to one or more muscles which increases muscle tone and causes movement. These sudden jerks are like those that occur in healthy people as they fall asleep.
- **Tonic-clonic seizures** (formerly called "grand mal") – begin with simultaneous loss of consciousness and the tonic phase (stiffening of the body). The person falls to the ground and often emits a loud cry as the chest muscles stiffen. Next comes the clonic phase, during which the muscles rhythmically jerk.

Partial Seizures

These seizures begin in a part of one hemisphere, generally in the temporal or frontal lobe. The two types of partial seizures, called simple and complex, are based on whether a person remains fully conscious during a seizure.

Simple

Complex

Main Forms of Partial Seizures

Simple partial seizures (sometimes called "auras"):
Seizure activity is focused in a specific area of the brain. A person remains alert and afterward is able to remember what happened. An aura or simple partial seizure may constitute the entire seizure or may precede a complex partial or generalized seizure. Symptoms vary depending on the area of the brain involved.

- Motor seizures cause a change in muscle activity and may involve jerking or stiffening of a part of the body.
- Sensory seizures may cause abnormal function in any of the five senses.
- Autonomic seizures affect involuntary functions and may cause a rapid heartbeat or breathing rate, sweating, or an unpleasant sensation in the abdomen, chest, throat or head.
- Psychic seizures may affect perception and memory or stimulate emotions such as fear.

Complex partial seizures:
Seizure is accompanied by impaired consciousness and recall. May also involve staring, automatic behaviors such as lip smacking, chewing, fumbling, picking, walking, grunting, repetition of words or phrases, or other symptoms and signs.

Diagnosing Epilepsy

There is no single test for epilepsy. The doctor will make a diagnosis based on a description of past seizures. Since those who have had a seizure are often unaware of what took place, the doctor may rely on others who witnessed the event. Details about how the patient felt before the attack and how it took place are very useful. The doctor will also review the patient's personal and family medical history, and will give a physical exam to check for other conditions that may have caused the attack.

There are tests designed to gather information about a patient's condition. The most commonly used test is an electroencephalogram (EEG). An EEG involves attaching a series of metal discs called electrodes to the patient's head to measure the brain's electrical activity. Most types of seizures are detectable with the EEG, but some abnormal activity may affect too small an area on the brain's surface or be located too deep to be detected. Other tests such as computed tomography (CT) and magnetic resonance imaging (MRI) can provide additional information about the brain. A doctor may order these tests to look for causes of the attack, such as a tumor, congenital malformation, or other changes in the brain.

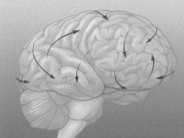

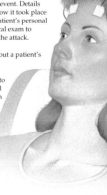

©2008 Wolters Kluwer | Lippincott Williams & Wilkins
Health

Published by **Anatomical Chart Company, Skokie, IL**

Migraines and Headaches

Vascular Headaches

The Pathways of a Migraine

A Migraine originates deep within the brain.

B Electrical impulses spread to other regions of the brain.

C Changes in nerve cell activity and blood flow may result in symptoms such as visual disturbance, numbness or tingling, and dizziness.

D Chemicals in the brain cause blood vessel dilation and inflammation of surrounding tissue.

E The inflammation irritates the trigeminal nerve, resulting in severe or throbbing pain.

Trigeminal nerve ganglion and nuclei

What Is a Vascular Headache?

A vascular headache is a condition that occurs when blood vessels in the brain dilate, triggering pain in the surrounding areas. Vascular headaches include **migraines** and **cluster headaches**.

Migraines are vascular headaches that occur on a more periodic basis, and they mainly affect women. They cause the senses to become more sensitive to change. A migraine is primarily an inherited disorder characterized by headaches ranging widely in intensity, frequency, and duration. The attacks are commonly felt only on one side and are usually associated with nausea, vomiting and loss of appetite. In some cases, the attacks are preceded by, or associated with, neurologic and mood disturbances.

Cluster headaches, as opposed to migraines, usually affect men more often than women. The attacks cause severe, one-sided pain, sometimes affecting the eye region and the area above it. They can also affect the temple regions along the side of the head. Cluster headaches usually occur in groups or series for 2 to 3 months. These attacks can last approximately 30 to 90 minutes and can occur from one to three times a day.

Vascular Theory for the Migraine

1. The hormone prostaglandin thromboxane is present in the blood stream. **(I)**

2. Hormone signals platelets to aggregate.

3. Platelet aggregation cause the release of serotonin (a chemical that transmits signals to nerves). **(II)**

4. Serotonin causes nerves to signal the blood vessels to vasoconstrict (decrease in diameter).

5. Vasoconstriction causes a decrease of blood flow around the brain (localized ischemia).

6. Localized ischemia causes an increase of acid (acidosis).

7. Localized ischemia and acidosis cause the non-innervated (no nerves) and innervated blood vessels to dilate (vasodilation).

8. Vasodilation of the innervated arteries results in headache phase. Perivascular inflammation (inflammation to surrounding vessels) may cause prolonged headache pain. Platelet aggregation decreases and therefore decreases the serotonin levels which results in vasodilation. A painful inflammation occurs around the surrounding areas which can persist into a postheadache phase. **(III)**

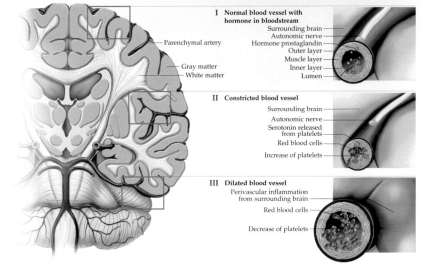

Parenchymal artery
Gray matter
White matter

I Normal blood vessel with hormone in bloodstream
Surrounding brain
Autonomic nerve
Hormone prostaglandin
Outer layer
Muscle layer
Inner layer
Lumen

II Constricted blood vessel
Surrounding brain
Autonomic nerve
Serotonin released from platelets
Red blood cells
Increase of platelets

III Dilated blood vessel
Perivascular inflammation from surrounding brain
Red blood cells
Decrease of platelets

Organic Headaches

Organic headaches may be due to a recent head injury or other disorder. Close observations should be made of those who have experienced a recent change in a headache pattern. The causes of these headaches include:

- Arteritis (inflammation of an artery)
- Infection
- Low cerebrospinal fluid (CSF) pressure
- Mass lesions such as:
  - Brain tumor
  - Hematoma (a swelling or mass of blood)
  - Cerebral hemorrhage
  - Cerebral edema
  - Aneurysm
  - Brain abscess

The following pattern is demonstrated in headaches resulting from a organic headache.

- Steady, non-throbbing, deep, dull ache.
- Exertion can trigger or exacerbate the headache.
- The frequency and duration will progressively increase.
- The headache can awaken the patient from a sound sleep.
- Pain can begin with a sudden, severe "thunderclap"-type headache.
- The headache is rarely as intense as the headache associated with a fever.
- The headache is steady, although it can be continuous in some patients.

Normal anatomy of the brain
Hematoma

Tension Headaches

*Temple: Temporalis muscle
*Forehead: Frontalis muscle

Tension-type headaches are characterized by a "hat band" or generalized pain over the entire head. The exact mechanism is still in dispute, but extreme muscle spasm and some dilation of the blood vessels are present. This category can be further divided into chronic and episodic. The distinguishing feature between these two types is the frequency of headaches.

- Chronic tension-type headaches occur at least 15 days per month for at least 6 months.
- Episodic is more common and occurs less frequent.

Chronic tension-type headache are sometimes called: chronic daily headache, coexisting migraine and tension headache, and transformed migraine. Chronic tension-type headaches are continuous or unremitting. Patients with these types of headaches usually have a long history of headaches. These headaches can sometimes be a manifestation of an underlying psychologic conflict.

Most people experiencing **episodic** tension-type headaches will use simple, over-the-counter analgesics to obtain relief.

Trapezius muscle
Levator scapulae muscle
*Back of the neck

*Areas involved in tension headaches

Headache Diagnostic Guide

	MIGRAINE	CLUSTER	TENSION-TYPE	ORGANIC
Frequency	2 to 8 times per month	1 to 3 times per day	Daily or almost daily	Varied
Duration	4 hours to 2 days, usually 12 to 18 hours	30 to 90 minutes	Constant	Varied
Onset	Gradual	Sudden, reaches peak of intensity in 1 to 3 minutes	Gradual	Varied, though onset of complaint may have been recent
Pain area	Unilateral. May switch sides or become bilateral.	Unilateral, usually periorbital	Bilateral, hatband	Unilateral
Characteristic pain	Throbbing, pulsating: moderate to severe	Steady, severe, excruciating, knife-like, sharp, probing	Steady, dull ache	Varied
Associated symptoms	Nausea or vomiting, diarrhea, sensitivity to senses and lightheadedness	Tearing of eye on same side as "runny nose"	None	Varied
Triggers	Stress, alcohol, missed meals menstruation and bright lights	Stress and alcohol	Stress, anxiety, fatigue depression	Head injury or disorder
Gender	3:1 female	10:1 male	Equal distribution	Equal distribution

Treatments

Medications are needed by some individuals. Your health care provider may prescribe one or more of the following medications:

Analgesics – These medications, such as aspirin, acetaminophen and ibuprofen may reduce the pain.

Triptans – a specific medication if taken during a migraine attack will either lessen or abort the headache.

Ergotamine preparations – These medications interfere with the widening of the blood vessels in the head and decrease the pain associated with migraines. Note: To enable your body to make the most use of the medication, it is important to take the medicine at the first sign of an attack.

Biofeedback – This type of treatment allows the person to regain control over the sometimes painful physiological reactions that would normally not be controllable. Your health care provider may refer you to a specialist in biofeedback therapy.

Other medications/treatments – Your health care provider may refer you to a specialist in the type of headache pain that you are having.

Healthy Lifestyle Changes

You may be able to decrease the chances of an attack. Here are some suggestions:

- Pay close attention to your diet.
- Regulate your sleep.
- Don't smoke.
- Avoid excess alcohol.
- Exercise regularly.
- Practice relaxation techniques.

It is very important to follow your health care provider's instructions and to take any medications as prescribed.

Understanding Multiple Sclerosis

Body of nerve cell

Axon

Normal myelin sheath around axon

Normal Nerve Cell

What Is Multiple Sclerosis?

Multiple sclerosis (MS) is an autoimmune disease, which means that the body's immune system attacks its own tissues. In MS, the immune system attacks the protective insulating layer known as the myelin sheath that surrounds the extensions of nerve cells in the brain and spinal cord. Myelin acts like an insulation on a wire. It allows the body to transmit electrical signals" rapidly from one nerve cell to another and over a long distance. Over time, as myelin is replaced with scar tissue (sclerosis), the brain's ability to transmit signals to the rest of the body is disrupted. The result may be a decrease or a complete loss of control of many neurological functions.

Symptoms & Signs

People with MS experience attacks of symptoms that can last from a few days to several months. These attacks are followed by periods of remission, or symptom-free phases. Early symptoms of MS may include:
• Feelings of tingling, burning, numbness, or pain.
• Double vision, blurry vision, or blindness.
• Weakness, dizziness, and fatigue.
During remission the patient may feel better, but there may be lingering stiffness, weakness, numbness, and vision problems. However, the disabilities (symptoms) may be more severe during relapse and include:
• Muscle spasms.
• Changes in bladder and bowel control.
• Slurred speech.
• Blindness.
• Sexual dysfunction.
• Paralysis.
• Confusion and forgetfulness.
Most people with MS do not develop the most severe symptoms, and regain enough function to continue to lead a normal life.

Prevention & Management

Currently there is no cure or prevention for MS. However, several drugs exist that can help manage symptoms and reduce the frequency of attacks. Additional therapies for managing symptoms include:
• Avoidance of heat– some sufferers may experience temporary worsening of symptoms with heat.
• Practice of healthy lifestyle to cope with fatigue and potential stress:
  • Getting enough rest.
  • Exercising regularly.
  • Eating a healthy, well-balanced diet with plenty of fiber.
  • Practicing relaxation techniques.

Types of Multiple Sclerosis

Benign multiple sclerosis
(Minimal to no accumulated disability (symptoms), few attacks, usually with return to normal between attacks)

Relapsing-Remitting multiple sclerosis
(No new disability (symptoms) between attacks)

Secondary Progressive multiple sclerosis
(Evolving from relapsing-remitting disease, there is a progressive disability (symptoms) with or without attacks)

Primary Progressive multiple sclerosis
(Steady increase in disability (symptoms) without attacks)

Increasing Disability

Time

Nerve Cell Affected by MS

Enlarged View of Nerve Fiber

Nerve fiber from within Central Nervous System

Axon part of nerve cell

Myelin sheath of nerve cell

Immune cells are involved in the destructive process of the myelin sheath

Myelin sheath damaged from multiple sclerosis

Exposed fiber

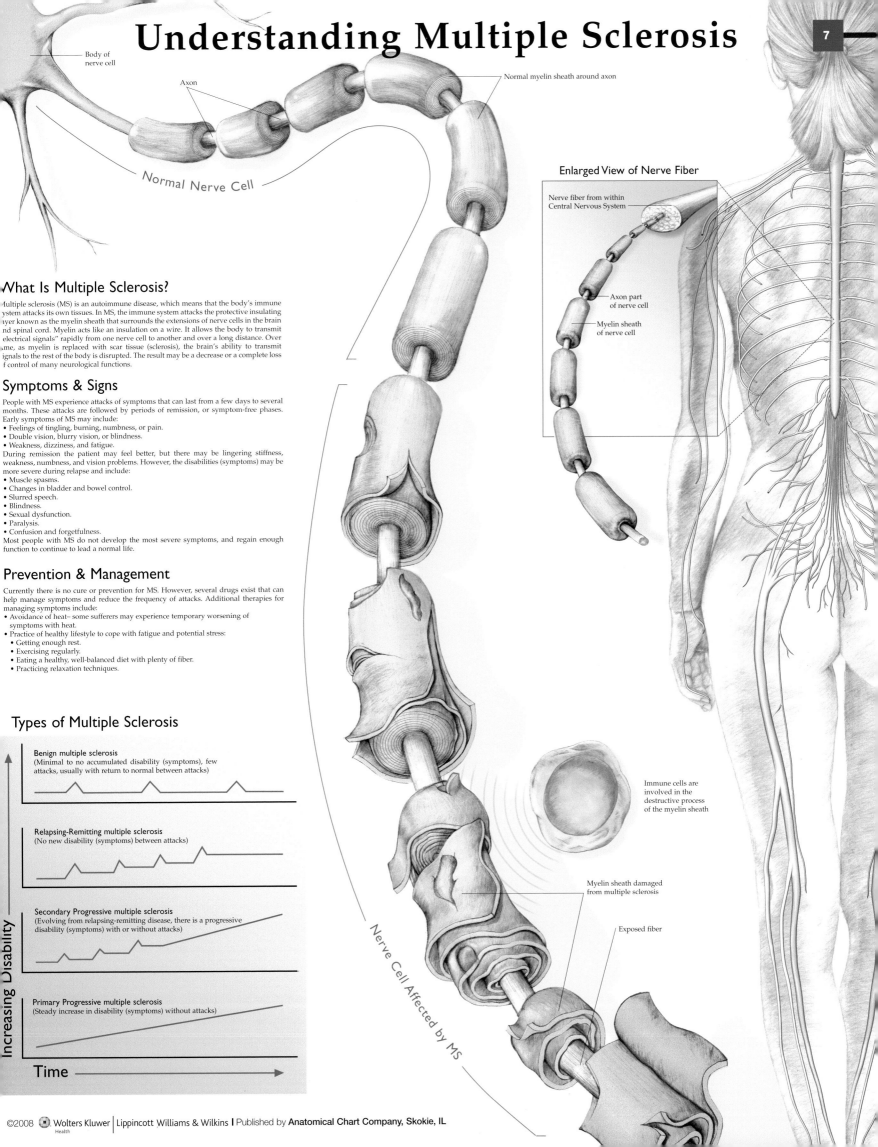

Understanding Pain

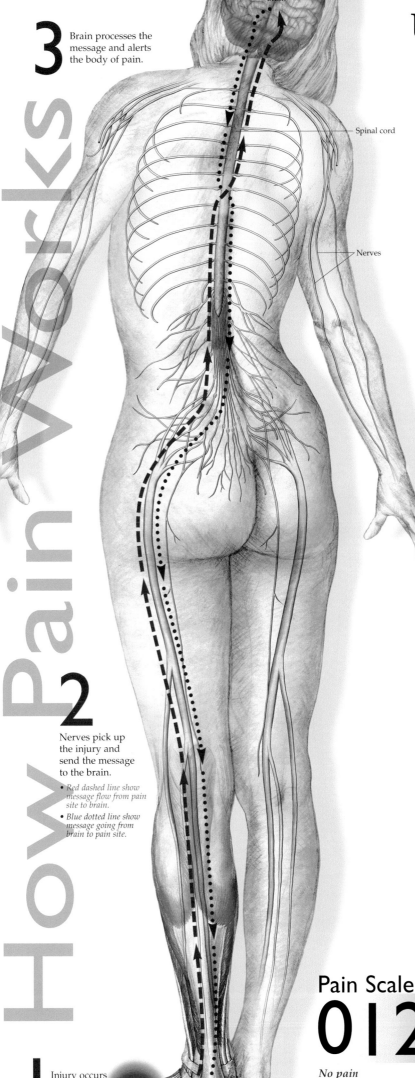

How Pain Works

3 Brain processes the message and alerts the body of pain.

Spinal cord

Nerves

2 Nerves pick up the injury and send the message to the brain.

- *Red dashed line show message flow from pain site to brain.*
- *Blue dotted line show message going from brain to pain site.*

1 Injury occurs in the body.

What Is Pain?

It is an unpleasant sensation occurring in varying degrees of severity associated with injury, disease, or emotional disorder.

2 Types of Pain

1. ACUTE PAIN

occurs as a result of injury to the body and generally disappears when the physical injury heals. Acute pain is linked to tissue injury. Anxiety is common with acute pain.

Examples include:
- Surgical pain
- Muscle strains
- Orthopedic-type injuries
- Labor and delivery

Symptoms: Patient is able to point to site of pain.
- Sharp
- Burning
- Cramping
- Aching
- Pressured

2. CHRONIC (PERSISTENT) PAIN

lasts beyond the normal healing period – usually at least 3 months. The pain may be multifocal and vague. There may be no signs on x-rays or scans to indicate the source of the pain since some pain may be generated by tissue injury. Depression is common with chronic pain.

Neuropathic chronic pain is a type of pain that is caused by injury to a nerve. Patients describe the pain as having tingling, numbness, or burning sensation. Neuropathic pain is difficult to treat.

Common types of neuropathic chronic pain include:
- Diabetic neuropathy – nerve damage as a result of high blood sugar.
- Post-herpetic neuralgia – pain from shingles after the blisters have healed.
- HIV/AIDS – pain from the viral illness or the drugs used to treat the disease.
- Peripheral vascular disease – pain in legs, usually during activity, from lack of blood supply to the extremities. The legs may be discolored, cold, and the skin may be shiny.

Symptoms:
- Painful itching
- Strange sensations
- Extreme sensitivity to normal touch and temperature
- Burning
- Electric-like sensation
- Painful numbness
- Pins and needles

Non-neuropathic chronic pain is pain that is not caused by injury to a nerve.

The most common types include:
- Low back pain – pain in the lower back from muscles, ligaments, tendons, arthritis, or damaged discs.
- Osteoarthritis – arthritis resulting from wear and tear of the joints and with normal aging.
- Rheumatoid arthritis – an autoimmune disorder resulting in pain, stiffness, and inflammation of the joints.

Symptoms: Poorly localized pain (patient may not be able to point to site of pain).
- Gnawing
- Pounding
- Deep aching

Unknown: There are many common chronic pain syndromes that are neither known to be chronic non-neuropathic nor neuropathic.

These include:
- Fibromyalgia syndrome – diffuse body pain with tenderness in the muscles.
- Tension headache – pressure-type headache lasting days to weeks and often not severe.
- Migraine headache – episodic headache that persists for hours to days with nausea and is often severe.
- Irritable bowel syndrome (IBS) – abdominal pain with cramping, bloating, and constipation often alternating with diarrhea.
- Some low back pain – back pain that is not muscular, not related to disc injury, and without a known cause.

Symptoms: May be a combination of chronic non-neuropathic and neuropathic symptoms.

Where do you Feel Pain?

Right   Left

Left   Right

Treatment

Specific treatment options need to be tailored to the individual patient. Be sure to consult with your healthcare professional to determine the right treatment for you.

Prevention techniques:
- Regular exercise   • Maintain a healthy body weight   • Use safe techniques when lifting heavy objects

Pain Scale

0 1 2 3 4 5 6 7 8 9 10

No pain

Rate your pain by choosing the number that best describes it.

Extreme pain

Understanding Parkinson's Disease

What is Parkinson's Disease?

Parkinson's Disease (PD) is a slowly progressive, degenerative disease of the brain. It affects nerve cells in areas of the brain called the basal ganglia and the substantia nigra. Nerve cells in the substantia nigra produce dopamine, a neurotransmitter that acts as a chemical messenger in brain circuits important for planning and controlling body movement. For reasons not yet understood, the nerve cells in the substantia nigra die. When 80% of dopamine is lost, symptoms such as tremor, slowness of movement, stiffness, and balance problems occur. PD usually occurs in men and women in their 60's, but can occur earlier. The cause of PD is largely unknown.

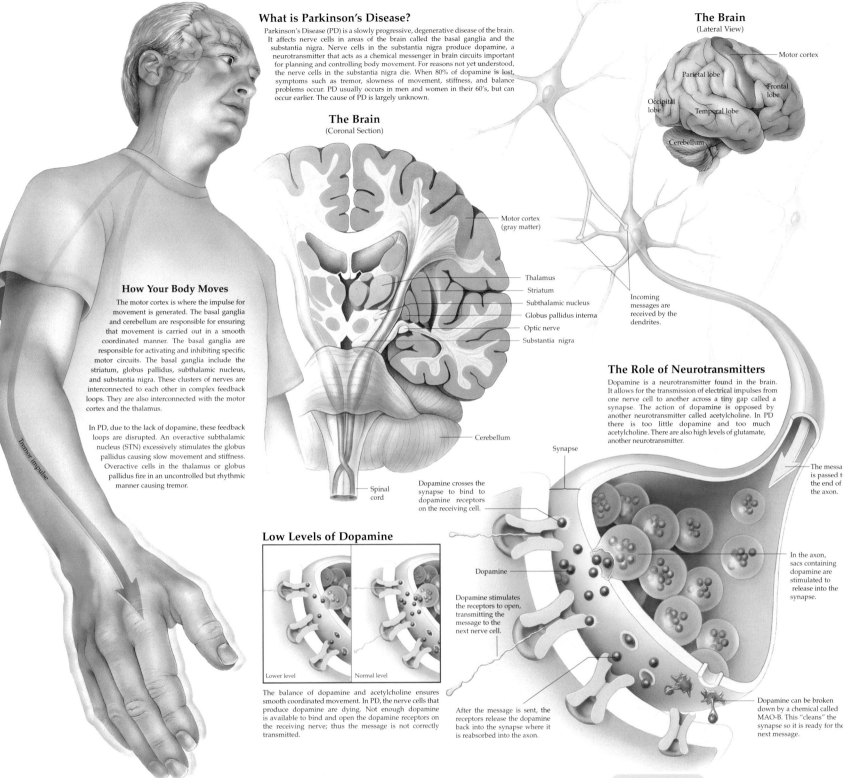

The Brain
(Coronal Section)

- Motor cortex (gray matter)
- Thalamus
- Striatum
- Subthalamic nucleus
- Globus pallidus interna
- Optic nerve
- Substantia nigra
- Cerebellum
- Spinal cord

The Brain
(Lateral View)

- Motor cortex
- Parietal lobe
- Frontal lobe
- Occipital lobe
- Temporal lobe
- Cerebellum

Incoming messages are received by the dendrites.

How Your Body Moves

The motor cortex is where the impulse for movement is generated. The basal ganglia and cerebellum are responsible for ensuring that movement is carried out in a smooth coordinated manner. The basal ganglia are responsible for activating and inhibiting specific motor circuits. The basal ganglia include the striatum, globus pallidus, subthalamic nucleus, and substantia nigra. These clusters of nerves are interconnected to each other in complex feedback loops. They are also interconnected with the motor cortex and the thalamus.

In PD, due to the lack of dopamine, these feedback loops are disrupted. An overactive subthalamic nucleus (STN) excessively stimulates the globus pallidus causing slow movement and stiffness. Overactive cells in the thalamus or globus pallidus fire in an uncontrolled but rhythmic manner causing tremor.

Tremor impulse

The Role of Neurotransmitters

Dopamine is a neurotransmitter found in the brain. It allows for the transmission of electrical impulses from one nerve cell to another across a tiny gap called a synapse. The action of dopamine is opposed by another neurotransmitter called acetylcholine. In PD there is too little dopamine and too much acetylcholine. There are also high levels of glutamate, another neurotransmitter.

- Synapse
- The message is passed to the end of the axon.
- Dopamine crosses the synapse to bind to dopamine receptors on the receiving cell.
- In the axon, sacs containing dopamine are stimulated to release into the synapse.
- Dopamine
- Dopamine stimulates the receptors to open, transmitting the message to the next nerve cell.
- Dopamine can be broken down by a chemical called MAO-B. This "cleans" the synapse so it is ready for the next message.

Low Levels of Dopamine

Lower level

Normal level

The balance of dopamine and acetylcholine ensures smooth coordinated movement. In PD, the nerve cells that produce dopamine are dying. Not enough dopamine is available to bind and open the dopamine receptors on the receiving nerve; thus the message is not correctly transmitted.

After the message is sent, the receptors release the dopamine back into the synapse where it is reabsorbed into the axon.

Medical Management

This is the first line of defense for PD patients. There are many options that may be used alone or in combination with each other to control symptoms.

1. Replace the missing dopamine in the brain. Levadopa enters the brain and is converted to dopamine. Carbidopa is used in combination to prevent breakdown of levadopa outside the brain which can cause nausea or irregularities of heart rhythm.

2. Optimize the delivery of levadopa to the brain by blocking COMT in the digestive system, allowing a steady supply of levadopa to reach the blood.

3. Block the breakdown of dopamine by MAO-B in the brain.

4. Introduce agents that mimic dopamine by binding to the dopamine receptors.

5. Reduce the activity of acetylcholine to bring the dopamine/acetylcholine activity in balance.

6. Block the excessive action of glutamate.

After a time on medication, patients may notice that each dose wears off before the next dose can be taken (wearing-off effect) or erratic fluctuations in dose effect (on-off effect). Another side effect patients may notice with time is dyskinesia, which are involuntary jerking or swaying movements of the body that typically occur at peak doses.

Surgical Management

When medical management fails due to fluctuations in the response, lack of effectiveness, or development of side effects such as dyskinesias, surgical options may be considered. These include destroying overactive areas of the brain or controlling them with electrical stimulation.

These procedures are done with a stereotactic frame attached to the skull. CT or MRI imaging is used to determine the exact location of the desired brain structure. Next, a small hole is made in the skull through which a probe is inserted into the brain structure.

- Probe
- Stereotactic frame

Pallidotomy

The internal part of the globus pallidus interna (GPi) is destroyed by passing a high-frequency energy current which heats it to a desired temperature. This procedure is useful in controlling dyskinesias.

Thalamotomy

The same energy current is used to destroy a small area in the thalamus. This procedure is useful in controlling tremor.

Deep-Brain Stimulation (DBS)

An electrode is implanted in the desired area of the brain (globus pallidus, thalamus, or subthalamus), and then connected to a pacemaker implanted under the skin below the collar bone. The pacemaker sends electrical signals to regulate activity. Thalamic stimulation controls tremor; GPi or STN stimulation controls slowness of movement.

Symptoms

Symptoms may vary from person to person as does the rate of progression. The most common symptoms are listed below.

- Bradykinesia: Slowness of movement, impaired dexterity, decreased blinking, drooling, lack of facial expression.
- Tremor: Involuntary shaking, more prominent in resting position and decreases with purposeful movement.
- Rigidity: stiffness caused by increase in muscle tone.
- Postural Instability: sense of imbalance, tendency to fall.

Other symptoms that may or may not occur:
- Freezing
- Shuffling gait
- Stooped posture
- Small handwriting
- Insomnia
- Depression

Many people with Parkinson's enjoy an active lifestyle and a normal life expectancy. As yet there is no cure or definitive way to slow disease progression. However it is an area of ongoing research with new treatments constantly being developed.

Resources & Support

Contact the American Parkinsons Disease Association at 800-223-2732 or the National Parkinson Foundation at 800-327-4545 or the Parkinson's Disease Foundation at 800-457-6676 for local support groups and informational booklets.

©2008 Wolters Kluwer | Lippincott Williams & Wilkins I Published by Anatomical Chart Company, Skokie, IL · Health

Understanding Sleep Disorders

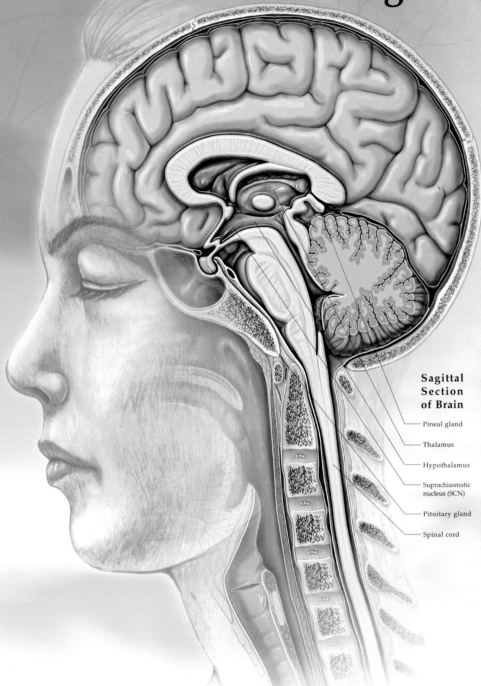

Sagittal Section of Brain

- Pineal gland
- Thalamus
- Hypothalamus
- Suprachiasmatic nucleus (SCN)
- Pituitary gland
- Spinal cord

What Is Sleep?

Sleep is a natural, reversible state of decreased responsiveness to the environment. During sleep, usually the eyes are closed and the body is relaxed and almost motionless. We think of sleep in contrast to wakefulness, when the body and mind are active. Although sleep provides important rest and restoration for the brain and body, the brain is very active during the portions of sleep when we are dreaming.

Why Does the Body Need Sleep?

Sleep is important for survival and appears to have specific functions for the endocrine, immune, cardiovascular, and nervous systems. It also has been suggested that sleep is important for bodily restoration, energy conservation, and memory consolidation. Not having an appropriate amount of normal, restful sleep may seriously affect daily functioning.

What Does the Suprachiasmatic Nucleus (SCN) Do?

The suprachiasmatic nucleus (SCN) is an area of the hypothalamus that initiates signals to other parts of the brain that control hormones, body temperature, and other functions that play a role in making you feel sleepy or wide awake. The SCN works like a biological clock that sets off a regulated pattern of activities that affect the whole body. The SCN controls the production of melatonin in the pineal gland. During the day the melatonin level is very low, but it increases in the evening and is elevated throughout the night, when you normally sleep. The functioning of the SCN normally helps you sleep for about 8 hours at night and remain awake for about 16 hours in the daytime and evening.

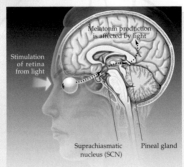

Melatonin production is affected by light

Stimulation of retina from light

Suprachiasmatic nucleus (SCN)

Pineal gland

Stages of Sleep

People usually cycle through different stages of sleep. Time spent in these stages may vary with age.

Non-REM *75–80% of sleep*	As you fall asleep, you enter non-REM sleep, which comprises of *Stages 1 – 4* *
*Stage 1 ***	Drowsiness and light sleep.
*Stage 2 ***	This stage takes up a majority of a night's total sleep. It is defined by unique EEG characteristics.
*Stages 3 & 4 ***	Deepest and most restorative sleep: Blood pressure drops, breathing slows down, and hormones are released for growth and development in youths.
REM *(Rapid Eye Movement)* *20–25% of sleep*	Occurs in episodes beginning about 90 minutes after onset of sleep and recurring with lengthening episodes about every 90 minutes. Most REM sleep is during the latter half of the night. The brain is active and dreams occur as the eyes dart back and forth. The body becomes relaxed and immobile. Breathing and heart rate may become irregular.

Normal Sleep Pattern

Awake
REM
Stage 1
2
3
4

Hours 1 2 3 4 5 6 7 8

Tips for a Good Night's Sleep

- Try to keep a regular bedtime and wakeup time.
- Avoid napping if you can't sleep well at night.
- Don't lie in bed awake if you can't sleep.
- Try to relax before going to bed.
- Exercise regularly, but not close to bedtime.
- Avoid caffeine, nicotine, and alcohol before bed.
- Maintain a comfortable room temperature.
- See a doctor if sleep problems continue.

Common Sleep Disorders

Sleep disorders can interfere with the ability to sleep or remain awake at the appropriate times. Some sleep disorders involve behaviors or experiences that occur in association with sleep. Some of the most common sleep disorders are shown below.

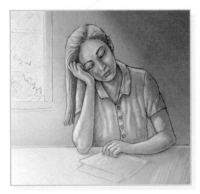

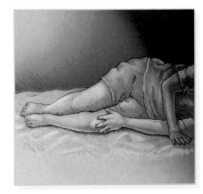

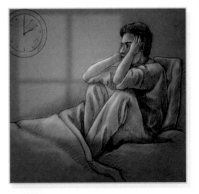

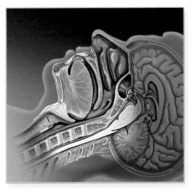

Narcolepsy

People with narcolepsy feel sleepy throughout their waking time, in spite of having sufficient opportunity for sleep at nighttime. They may nap several times a day but feel refreshed only for short periods. At times, sleep seems irresistible. They often have problems concentrating. Inattention and sleepiness can interfere with normal daily functioning. People with narcolepsy may experience cataplexy (*sudden muscle weakness during emotional situations*) and, when falling asleep, a brief sense of muscle paralysis or dreamlike hallucinations.

Restless Legs Syndrome (RLS)

Restless legs syndrome (RLS) is a disorder that causes a very unpleasant crawling sensation, mostly in the legs. The natural response is an urge to move them for relief. It usually is worst in the evening and when someone is at rest. It often interferes with the ability to sleep and may cause involuntary kicking during sleep. Someone with severe RLS may feel very uncomfortable sitting for a prolonged period of time in a theater or riding long distances in a car. Restless legs syndrome symptoms can begin at any age.

Insomnia

Insomnia is the most common sleep problem. It may include difficulty falling asleep and staying asleep, as well as a sense of light or unrefreshing sleep. Most commonly it is due to stress, but it also may result from psychiatric (*mental*), medical, and other sleep problems. Poor sleep habits can contribute to insomnia. For most people, insomnia lasts just a few days or weeks, but for others it may be a chronic condition lasting years. The daytime consequences are fatigue, lack of energy, difficulty concentrating, and irritability.

Obstructive Sleep Apnea

Obstructive sleep apnea is a recurrent interruption in breathing during sleep. It results from sleep-related muscle relaxation in the upper airway, which leads to a decrease or complete blockage of airflow for brief periods. The blood oxygen level may fall, causing arousals or awakenings that can disturb sleep. People with severe sleep apnea may be dangerously sleepy during the daytime. Those who are obese or snore loudly are at the greatest risk for sleep apnea, but others may have sleep apnea due to large tonsils or other features of their airway anatomy.

©2008 Wolters Kluwer Health | Lippincott Williams & Wilkins | Published by Anatomical Chart Company, Skokie, IL

Understanding Stroke

What Is Stroke?

Stroke refers to the sudden death of brain tissue caused by a lack of oxygen resulting from an interrupted blood supply. An **infarct** is the area of the brain that has "died" because of this lack of oxygen. There are two ways that brain tissue death can occur. **Ischemic stroke** is a blockage or reduction of blood flow in an artery that feeds that area of the brain. It is the most common cause of an infarct. **Hemorrhagic stroke** results from bleeding within and around the brain causing compression and tissue injury.

Ischemic Stroke

This type of stroke results from a blockage or reduction of blood flow to an area of the brain. This blockage may result from atherosclerosis and blood clot formation.

Atherosclerosis is the deposit of cholesterol and plaque within the walls of arteries. These deposits may become large enough to narrow the lumen and reduce the flow of blood while also causing the artery to lose its ability to stretch.

A **thrombus**, or blood clot, forms on the roughened surface of atherosclerotic plaques that develop in the wall of the artery. The thrombus can enlarge and eventually block the lumen of the artery.

Lumen
Plaque
Thrombus

Common Sites of Plaque Formation
(Indicated by yellow circles)

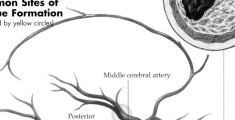

Middle cerebral artery

Posterior cerebral artery

Anterior cerebral artery

Anterior inferior cerebellar artery

Posterior inferior cerebellar artery

Embolus

Internal carotid artery

Embolus

Vertebral artery

Common carotid artery

Part of a thrombus may break off and become an **embolus**. An embolus travels through the blood stream until it reaches a vessel too small for it to pass through, thus blocking it.

Emboli commonly come from the heart, where different diseases can cause thrombus formation.

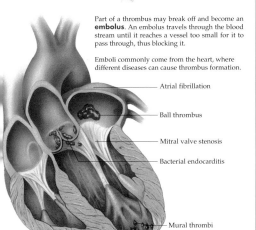

Atrial fibrillation

Ball thrombus

Mitral valve stenosis

Bacterial endocarditis

Mural thrombi

Myocardial infarction

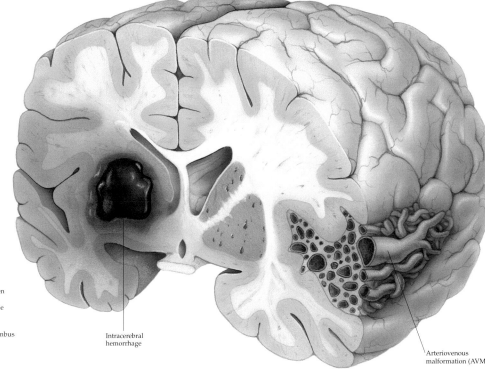

Intracerebral hemorrhage

Arteriovenous malformation (AVM)

Hemorrhagic Stroke

This type of stroke is caused by bleeding within and around the brain. Bleeding that fills the spaces between the brain and the skull is called a **subarachnoid hemorrhage**. It is caused by ruptured aneurysms, arteriovenous malformations, and head trauma. Bleeding within the brain tissue itself is known as **intracerebral hemorrhage** and is primarily caused by hypertension.

An **aneurysm** is a weakening of the arterial wall that causes it to stretch and balloon. It usually occurs where the artery branches.

Hypertension is an elevation of blood pressure that may cause tiny arterioles to burst causing the tissue beyond the rupture to die. Blood vessels in the dead tissue then leak causing more bleeding.

Circle of Willis

Aneurysm

An **arteriovenous malformation** (AVM) is an abnormality of the brain's blood vessels in which arteries lead directly into veins without first going through a capillary bed. The pressure of the blood coming through the arteries is too high for the veins, causing them to dilate in order to transport the higher volume of blood. AVM's may burst and also cause symptoms by putting pressure on sensitive areas causing seizures, or pain.

Microaneurysm

Arterioles

Subarachnoid hemorrhage

Normal Functional Areas of Brain

The brain has two sides: a right hemisphere that controls the left side of the body and a left hemisphere that controls the right side of the body. Each hemisphere has four lobes and a cerebellum that control our daily functions. Depending on what part of the brain has been affected, stroke victims experience a variety of neurological deficits. Rehabilitation is crucial to the stroke patient's recovery. Physical therapists and speech therapists help patients "relearn" their lost functions and devise ways to cope with the loss of those they cannot regain.

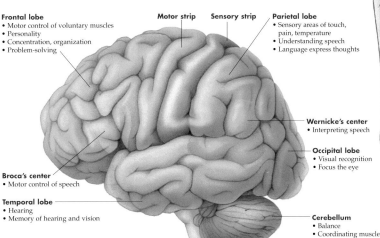

Frontal lobe
• Motor control of voluntary muscles
• Personality
• Concentration, organization
• Problem-solving

Motor strip   Sensory strip

Parietal lobe
• Sensory areas of touch, pain, temperature
• Understanding speech
• Language express thoughts

Wernicke's center
• Interpreting speech

Occipital lobe
• Visual recognition
• Focus the eye

Broca's center
• Motor control of speech

Temporal lobe
• Hearing
• Memory of hearing and vision

Cerebellum
• Balance
• Coordinating muscle movement

Brain stem
• Controls heart rate and rate of breathing

Events Leading to Stroke

Stroke victims often have small strokes or "warning signs," before a large permanent attack.

Transient Ischemic Attacks (TIAs) are brief attacks that last anywhere from a few minutes to 24 hours. The symptoms resolve completely and the person returns to normal. It is possible to have several TIAs before a large attack.

Complete Infarction (CI) is an attack that leaves permanent tissue death and results in serious neurological deficits. Recovery is usually not total and takes longer than three weeks.

Common Neurological Deficits After Stroke

Left-sided stroke
• Right-sided paralysis
• Speech/language deficits
• Slow, cautious behavior
• Hemianopsia of right visual field
• Memory loss in language
• Right-sided dysarthria
• Aphasia
• Apraxia

Right-sided stroke
• Left-sided paralysis
• Spatial/perceptual deficits
• Quick, impulsive behavior
• Hemianopsia of left visual field
• Memory loss in performance
• Left-sided dysarthria

Related Terms

Paralysis - Loss of muscle function and sensation
Hemiparesis - Weakness of muscles on one side of body
Hemianopsia - Loss of sight in half of visual field
Aphasia - Difficulty with oral communication, reduced ability to read or write
Apraxia - Inability to control muscles; movement is uncoordinated and jerky
Dysarthria - Slurring of speech and "mouth droop" on one side of face due to muscle weakness

Risks for Stroke

Hypertension
Heart disease
Atherosclerosis
Previous TIAs
High cholesterol
High alcohol consumption
Obesity
Diabetes
Bruit noise in carotid artery
Cigarette smoking
Oral contraceptive use
Family history of stroke

©2008 Wolters Kluwer Health | Lippincott Williams & Wilkins | Published by Anatomical Chart Company, Skokie, IL

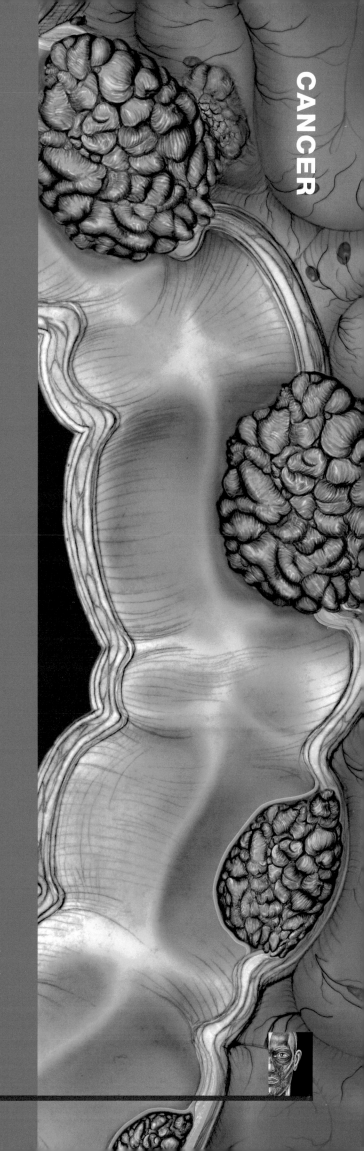

CANCER

Understanding Cancer

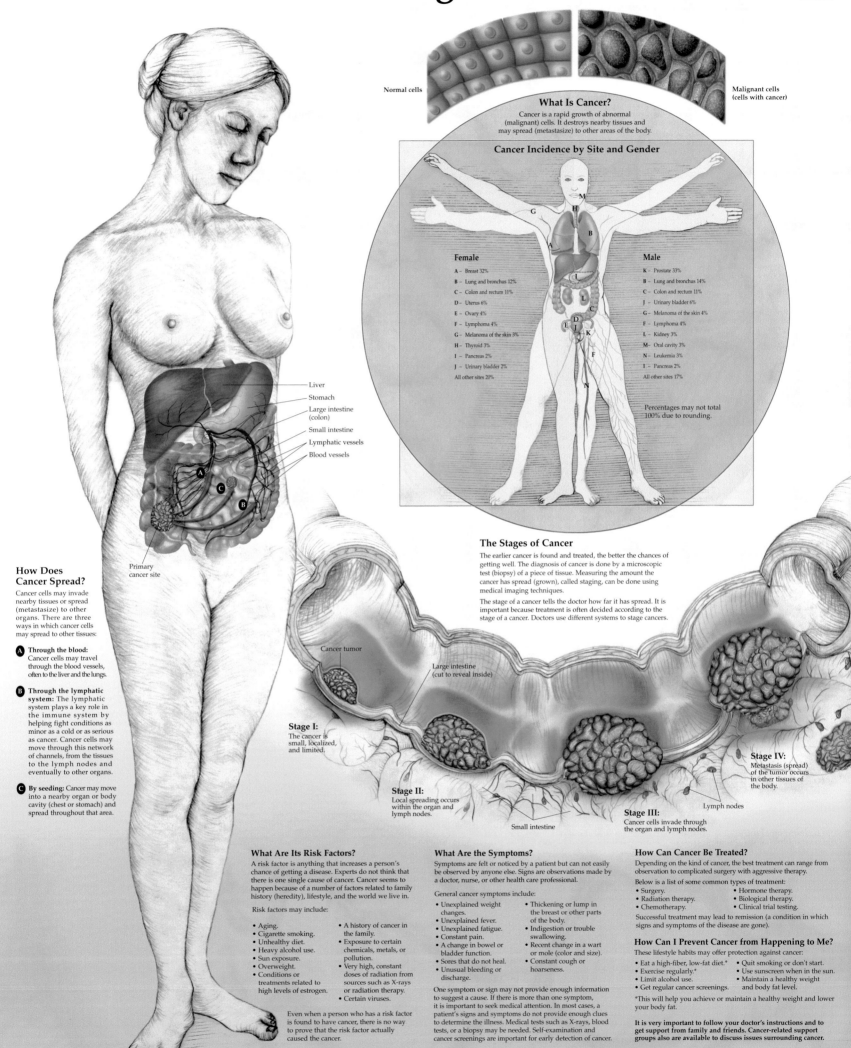

Normal cells

Malignant cells (cells with cancer)

What Is Cancer?
Cancer is a rapid growth of abnormal (malignant) cells. It destroys nearby tissues and may spread (metastasize) to other areas of the body.

Cancer Incidence by Site and Gender

Female
A – Breast 32%
B – Lung and bronchus 12%
C – Colon and rectum 11%
D – Uterus 6%
E – Ovary 4%
F – Lymphoma 4%
G – Melanoma of the skin 3%
H – Thyroid 3%
I – Pancreas 2%
J – Urinary bladder 2%
All other sites 20%

Male
K – Prostate 33%
B – Lung and bronchus 14%
C – Colon and rectum 11%
J – Urinary bladder 6%
G – Melanoma of the skin 4%
F – Lymphoma 4%
L – Kidney 3%
M– Oral cavity 3%
N – Leukemia 3%
I – Pancreas 2%
All other sites 17%

Percentages may not total 100% due to rounding.

Liver
Stomach
Large intestine (colon)
Small intestine
Lymphatic vessels
Blood vessels
Primary cancer site

How Does Cancer Spread?
Cancer cells may invade nearby tissues or spread (metastasize) to other organs. There are three ways in which cancer cells may spread to other tissues:

A Through the blood: Cancer cells may travel through the blood vessels, often to the liver and the lungs.

B Through the lymphatic system: The lymphatic system plays a key role in the immune system by helping fight conditions as minor as a cold or as serious as cancer. Cancer cells may move through this network of channels, from the tissues to the lymph nodes and eventually to other organs.

C By seeding: Cancer may move into a nearby organ or body cavity (chest or stomach) and spread throughout that area.

The Stages of Cancer
The earlier cancer is found and treated, the better the chances of getting well. The diagnosis of cancer is done by a microscopic test (biopsy) of a piece of tissue. Measuring the amount the cancer has spread (grown), called staging, can be done using medical imaging techniques.

The stage of a cancer tells the doctor how far it has spread. It is important because treatment is often decided according to the stage of a cancer. Doctors use different systems to stage cancers.

Cancer tumor

Large intestine (cut to reveal inside)

Stage I: The cancer is small, localized, and limited.

Stage II: Local spreading occurs within the organ and lymph nodes.

Small intestine

Stage III: Cancer cells invade through the organ and lymph nodes.

Lymph nodes

Stage IV: Metastasis (spread) of the tumor occurs in other tissues of the body.

What Are Its Risk Factors?
A risk factor is anything that increases a person's chance of getting a disease. Experts do not think that there is one single cause of cancer. Cancer seems to happen because of a number of factors related to family history (heredity), lifestyle, and the world we live in.

Risk factors may include:

- Aging.
- Cigarette smoking.
- Unhealthy diet.
- Heavy alcohol use.
- Sun exposure.
- Overweight.
- Conditions or treatments related to high levels of estrogen.
- A history of cancer in the family.
- Exposure to certain chemicals, metals, or pollution.
- Very high, constant doses of radiation from sources such as X-rays or radiation therapy.
- Certain viruses.

Even when a person who has a risk factor is found to have cancer, there is no way to prove that the risk factor actually caused the cancer.

What Are the Symptoms?
Symptoms are felt or noticed by a patient but can not easily be observed by anyone else. Signs are observations made by a doctor, nurse, or other health care professional.

General cancer symptoms include:

- Unexplained weight changes.
- Unexplained fever.
- Unexplained fatigue.
- Constant pain.
- A change in bowel or bladder function.
- Sores that do not heal.
- Unusual bleeding or discharge.
- Thickening or lump in the breast or other parts of the body.
- Indigestion or trouble swallowing.
- Recent change in a wart or mole (color and size).
- Constant cough or hoarseness.

One symptom or sign may not provide enough information to suggest a cause. If there is more than one symptom, it is important to seek medical attention. In most cases, a patient's signs and symptoms do not provide enough clues to determine the illness. Medical tests such as X-rays, blood tests, or a biopsy may be needed. Self-examination and cancer screenings are important for early detection of cancer.

How Can Cancer Be Treated?
Depending on the kind of cancer, the best treatment can range from observation to complicated surgery with aggressive therapy.

Below is a list of some common types of treatment:
- Surgery.
- Radiation therapy.
- Chemotherapy.
- Hormone therapy.
- Biological therapy.
- Clinical trial testing.

Successful treatment may lead to remission (a condition in which signs and symptoms of the disease are gone).

How Can I Prevent Cancer from Happening to Me?
These lifestyle habits may offer protection against cancer:
- Eat a high-fiber, low-fat diet.*
- Exercise regularly.*
- Limit alcohol use.
- Get regular cancer screenings.
- Quit smoking or don't start.
- Use sunscreen when in the sun.
- Maintain a healthy weight and body fat level.

*This will help you achieve or maintain a healthy weight and lower your body fat.

It is very important to follow your doctor's instructions and to get support from family and friends. Cancer-related support groups also are available to discuss issues surrounding cancer.

Understanding Breast Cancer

What Is Breast Cancer?

Breast cancer is the most common form of cancer in women and is the number two killer (after lung cancer) of women age 35 to 54. It can also occur in men, though incidence is rare. The survival rate has improved because of earlier diagnosis and the variety of treatments now available. Most breast cancer occurs in the upper outer quadrant (the upper part of the breast closest to the arm). A woman may not be able to feel a slow-growing breast tumor by touch for up to eight years, until it is 1-centimeter in diameter. Breast cancer may spread by way of the lymphatic system or bloodstream to the lungs, liver, bones and other organs, or directly to the skin or surrounding tissues.

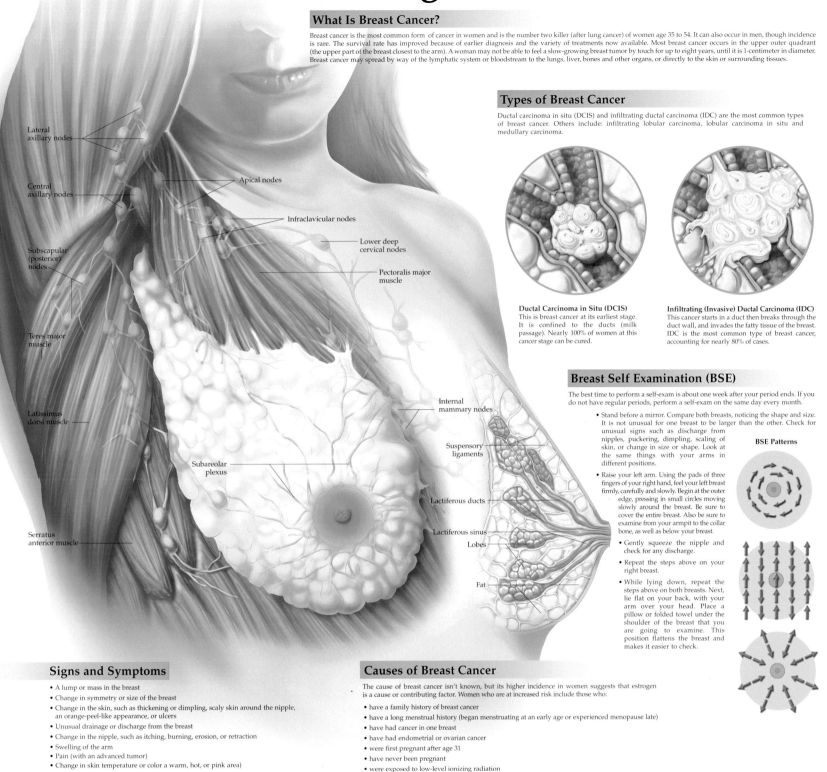

Types of Breast Cancer

Ductal carcinoma in situ (DCIS) and infiltrating ductal carcinoma (IDC) are the most common types of breast cancer. Others include: infiltrating lobular carcinoma, lobular carcinoma in situ and medullary carcinoma.

Ductal Carcinoma in Situ (DCIS)
This is breast cancer at its earliest stage. It is confined to the ducts (milk passage). Nearly 100% of women at this cancer stage can be cured.

Infiltrating (Invasive) Ductal Carcinoma (IDC)
This cancer starts in a duct then breaks through the duct wall, and invades the fatty tissue of the breast. IDC is the most common type of breast cancer, accounting for nearly 80% of cases.

Breast Self Examination (BSE)

The best time to perform a self-exam is about one week after your period ends. If you do not have regular periods, perform a self-exam on the same day every month.

- Stand before a mirror. Compare both breasts, noticing the shape and size. It is not unusual for one breast to be larger than the other. Check for unusual signs such as discharge from nipples, puckering, dimpling, scaling of skin, or change in size or shape. Look at the same things with your arms in different positions.
- Raise your left arm. Using the pads of three fingers of your right hand, feel your left breast firmly, carefully and slowly. Begin at the outer edge, pressing in small circles moving slowly around the breast. Be sure to cover the entire breast. Also be sure to examine from your armpit to the collar bone, as well as below your breast.
- Gently squeeze the nipple and check for any discharge.
- Repeat the steps above on your right breast.
- While lying down, repeat the steps above on both breasts. Next, lie flat on your back, with your arm over your head. Place a pillow or folded towel under the shoulder of the breast that you are going to examine. This position flattens the breast and makes it easier to check.

BSE Patterns

Signs and Symptoms

- A lump or mass in the breast
- Change in symmetry or size of the breast
- Change in the skin, such as thickening or dimpling, scaly skin around the nipple, an orange-peel-like appearance, or ulcers
- Unusual drainage or discharge from the breast
- Change in the nipple, such as itching, burning, erosion, or retraction
- Swelling of the arm
- Pain (with an advanced tumor)
- Change in skin temperature or color a warm, hot, or pink area

Causes of Breast Cancer

The cause of breast cancer isn't known, but its higher incidence in women suggests that estrogen is a cause or contributing factor. Women who are at increased risk include those who:

- have a family history of breast cancer
- have a long menstrual history (began menstruating at an early age or experienced menopause late)
- have had cancer in one breast
- have had endometrial or ovarian cancer
- were first pregnant after age 31
- have never been pregnant
- were exposed to low-level ionizing radiation

Staging

Clinical staging is a part of the pretreatment evaluation and is performed by histologic examination of the biopsied tissue and axillary specimen to assess the extent of the disease, lymph node involvement, the status of the other breast, and the possibility of systemic metastasis (passing from one site to another).
The most commonly used system is the **Tumor-Nodes-Metastasis system (TNM)**. T represents the primary tumor, N describes lymph node involvement, and M describes metastasis, if any.

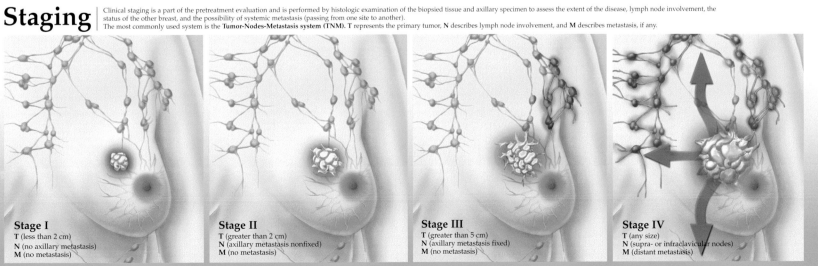

Stage I
T (less than 2 cm)
N (no axillary metastasis)
M (no metastasis)

Stage II
T (greater than 2 cm)
N (axillary metastasis nonfixed)
M (no metastasis)

Stage III
T (greater than 5 cm)
N (axillary metastasis fixed)
M (no metastasis)

Stage IV
T (any size)
N (supra- or infraclavicular nodes)
M (distant metastasis)

Fallopian Tube

Uterus

Fallopian Tube

Ovary

Ovary

Body of Uterus

Understanding Cervical Cancer

The cervix is the lower, narrow end of the uterus. Cervical cancer is a disease in which cancer cells form in the tissues of the cervix. The most common types of cervical cancers are squamous cell cancer, adenosquamous cancer, and adenocarcinoma.

THE CERVIX AS VIEWED THROUGH A SPECULUM ON A PELVIC EXAM

Cervix

Ectocervical lesion

Vaginal wall

RISK FACTORS

Persistent human papilloma virus (HPV) infection, a sexually-transmitted disease, is the major risk factor for developing cervical cancer. Other risk factors include:
- Smoking cigarettes
- History of sexually-transmitted disease
- Many sexual partners
- First sexual intercourse at a young age
- Multiple children (Multiparous)
- Long-term use of oral contraceptives
- Weakened immune system

SIGNS AND SYMPTOMS

There are usually no signs or symptoms early in the disease, although cervical cancer can be detected with yearly check-ups.
Some possible signs, which may appear as the disease progresses, include:
- **Abnormal vaginal bleeding** (bleeding between periods, after intercourse, or after menopause)
- **Unusual vaginal discharge** (may be pale, watery, red, or foul-smelling)
- **Pelvic pain at rest or during intercourse**

Note: many other conditions may cause these same symptoms.

DIAGNOSIS / SCREENING

Tests that are used to detect and diagnose cervical cancer include:
- **Pelvic exam:** The doctor uses a speculum to visually examine the cervix and one or two fingers to feel for abnormalities.
- **Pap smear:** Cells from the cervix and vagina is collected and examined under a microscope to identify any abnormalities.
- **Colposcopy:** A colposcope, an instrument with a magnifying lens, is used to examine the vagina and cervix more closely.
- **Biopsy:** If abnormalities are found on colposcopy, a sample of tissue from the cervix is taken to view under a microscope.
- **Endocervical curettage:** Cells from the cervical canal is collected using a spoon-shaped instrument called a curette.
- **Cone biopsy (conization):** A cautery loop or a scalpel is used to remove the outer part of the cervix; this may also cure very early stage cervical cancer.

TREATMENT

Treatment options depend on the following:
- Stage of the cancer
- Size of the tumor
- Patient's desire to have children
- Patient's age and other medical problems

Treatment options include:
- **Surgery:** an operation to remove cancer; may include radical hysterectomy or more limited procedures to preserve fertility in very early stage cancer.
- **Radiation therapy:** use of high-energy x-rays or other types of radiation to kill cancer cells.
- **Chemotherapy:** use of drugs to stop the growth of cancer cells, either by killing the cells or by stopping the cells from dividing.

Two or more methods may be used to treat cervical cancer in the same patient.

DETECTED EARLY, CERVICAL CANCER HAS A BETTER CHANCE TO BE CURED.

PREVENTION

- Having yearly checkups, including pap smear exam.
  – HPV testing may be helpful for some pap smear abnormalities and in women over age 30.
  – For patients who have had cervical cancer in the past, your doctor may recommend more frequent testing for the first few years after treatment.
- Talking to your doctor about a HPV vaccination. To be most effective, vaccination should occur before becoming sexually active.
- The risks of developing cervical cancer can be reduced by:
  – Regular pelvic and pap smear exams
  – Limiting the number of sexual partners
  – Avoiding sex with people who have had multiple sexual partners
  – Delaying the date of first sexual intercourse
  – Not smoking
  – HPV vaccination in appropriate patients

CARCINOMA IN SITU

Normal cells

Pre-malignant cells

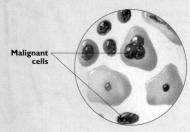

SQUAMOUS CELL CARCINOMA

Malignant cells

STAGING

After the cervical cancer is diagnosed, the stage of the cancer (how far the cancer has spread) is determined. The following stages are used for cervical cancer:

STAGE 0: (Carcinoma in Situ): Cancer is found only in the outer layer of cells lining the cervix.
STAGE I: Cancer has invaded past the surface layer, but is found only in the cervix.
STAGE II: Cancer has spread beyond the cervix but not to the pelvic wall nor to the lower third of the vagina.
STAGE III: Cancer has extended to the lower third of the vagina; it may have spread to the pelvic wall and/or blocked kidney functions.
STAGE IV: Cancer has spread to the bladder, rectum or other parts of the body.

Common tests used to determine the stage of the cancer include:
- Pelvic exam
- Imaging tests:
  – X-rays of the chest and urinary system
  – Barium enema to assess the rectum
Additional tests used to determine treatment options include:
- CT scan (CAT scan) – Computerized tomography or computerized axial tomography
- MRI – Magnetic resonance imaging
- PET scan – Positron emission tomography

STAGE 0 - I

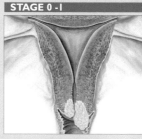

Carcinoma confined to the cervix.

Carcinoma confined to the cervix, "cauliflower" lesion.

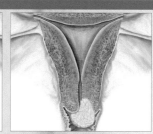

Bulky endocervical barrel-shaped lesion.

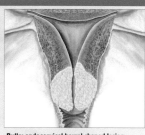

STAGE 2

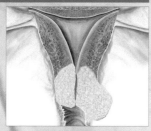

Carcinoma extends into the upper vagina.

Carcinoma extends into the parametrium (fibrous tissue that separates the cervix from the bladder), but does not extend to the pelvic sidewall.

STAGE 3

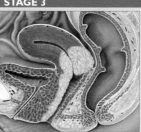

Carcinoma involves the anterior (front) vaginal wall, extending to the lower third of the vagina.

The parametrium is completely invaded and the carcinoma extends to the pelvic sidewall.

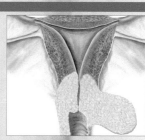

STAGE 4

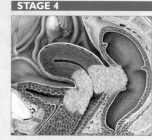

The bladder base or rectum is involved; distant metastasis may also be present.

Understanding Colorectal Cancer

Transverse colon

Adenocarcinoma of colon

Circumferencial carcinoma of transverse colon

Ascending colon

Cecum

Adenocarcinoma of jejunum

Colonic polyps

Vermiform appendix

Descending colon

Adenocarcinoma of rectosigmoid region

Rectum

Anus

Sigmoid colon

What is Colorectal Cancer? Cancer that begins in the colon is called colon cancer and cancer that begins in the rectum is called rectal cancer. Cancers affecting either of these organs is also called colorectal cancer.

Colorectal cancer occurs when some of the cells that line the colon or the rectum become abnormal and grow out of control. The abnormal growing cells create a tumor, which is the cancer.

Who is at Risk for Colorectal Cancer? Everybody is at risk for colorectal cancer. Colorectal cancer is the 2nd leading type of cancer causing deaths in the U.S.A. The majority of people who develop colorectal cancer have no known risk factors.

The exact cause of colorectal cancer is not yet known. Below are some factors that could increase a person's risk of developing this disease.

- **Age** - The disease is more common in people over 50. The chance of getting colorectal cancer increases with each decade of life. However, it has also been detected in younger people.
- **Gender** - Overall the risks are equal, but women have a higher risk for colon cancer and men are more likely to develop rectal cancer.
- **Polyps** - Begin as non-cancerous growths on the inner wall of the colon or rectum; this is fairly common in people over 50 years of age. Adenomas are one type of non-cancerous polyps that can mutate and are the potential precursors of colon and rectal cancer.
- **Personal history** - Research shows that women who have a history of ovarian or uterine cancer have a slight increased risk of developing colorectal cancer. In addition, people who have Ulcerative colitis or Crohn's disease also are at higher risk.
- **Family history** - Parents, siblings, and children of a person who has had colorectal cancer are more likely to develop the disease themselves. A family history of familial polyposis, adenomatous polyps, or hereditary polyp syndrome also increases the risk.
- **Diet** - A diet high in fat and calories and low in fiber may be linked to a greater risk.
- **Lifestyle factors** - Alcohol, smoking, lack of exercise, and overweight status are additional risk factors.
- **Diabetes** - Diabetics have a 30-40% increased risk.

Signs & Symptoms

Colorectal cancer may not cause any symptoms in early stages. However the following signs should raise suspicion:

- Change in bowel habits: Diarrhea or constipation or a change in the consistency of stool
- Narrow, pencil-thin stools
- Rectal bleed or blood in stool
- Persistent abdominal discomfort such as gas, pain or cramps
- Feeling bowel does not empty completely
- Unexplained weight loss
- Constant fatigue

Screening tests

- **Fecal Occult Blood Test (FOBT)** - Checks for hidden blood in the stool.
- **Sigmoidoscopy** - Sigmoidoscope is a long, flexible tube with a tiny video camera at the tip that is inserted into the rectum to allow the doctor to view the lower part of the colon – the rectum, the descending colon, and the sigmoid colon.
- **Colonoscopy** - Colonoscope is a long, flexible tube with a tiny video camera at the tip that is inserted into the rectum to allow the doctor to view the inside of the entire colon. The doctor may also biopsy the tissue and remove polyps during a colonoscopy.
- **Barium enema** - Chalky white liquid called barium is released into the colon (through the rectum) and then an X-ray is performed.
- **Digital rectal exam**

Diagnostic tests

If the screening tests or symptoms indicate the possibility of colorectal cancer, patients will undergo a diagnostic workup. These will help determine if colorectal cancer is present and the stage of the disease. Tests may include:

- **Medical history**
- **Physical exam**
- **Blood tests**
- **Biopsy** - abnormal tissue is removed and examined during a screening test to check for cancer cells.
- **Imaging Tests**
- **Ultrasound**
- **Computed tomography (CT)**
- **Magnetic resonance imaging (MRI)**
- **Chest X-ray** (to see if the cancer has spread to the lungs)

Treatments

Choice of treatment(s) depends on the location of the tumor (colon or rectum) and the stage of the disease. Common types of treatments include:

- **Surgery** - This is the most common treatment. It is used for removal of polyps and tumors and to check for the spread of the disease. Common types include laparoscopy and open surgery. After removal of part of the colon or rectum, the healthy parts are usually reconnected. When reconnection is not possible, a colostomy may be performed.
- **Chemotherapy** - Drug therapy that prevents the spread of cancer cells.
- **Radiation Therapy** - Also known as Radiotherapy, uses high energy-rays to kill cancer cells.
- **Biological Therapy** - Patients receive a monoclonal antibody through a vein which binds to colorectal cancer cells, interfering with their cell growth and spread in the body.

The Stages of Cancer

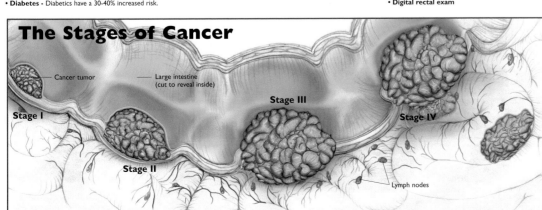

Cancer tumor

Large intestine (cut to reveal inside)

Stage I

Stage II

Stage III

Stage IV

Lymph nodes

The earlier cancer is found and treated, the better the chances of getting well. The diagnosis of cancer is made by a microscopic test (biopsy) of a piece of tissue. Medical imaging techniques are used to measure how much the cancer has spread (grown) – this is known as staging. The doctors often decide on the treatment based on the stage of cancer.

Doctors identify the stages of cancer as follows:

Stage I: The cancer has grown into the inner wall of the colon or rectum. The tumor has not yet reached the outer wall of the colon or extended outside the colon. Dukes' A is another name for Stage I colorectal cancer.

Stage II: The tumor extends more deeply into or through the wall of the colon or rectum. It may have invaded nearby tissue, but cancer cells have not yet spread to the lymph nodes. Dukes' B is another name for Stage II colorectal cancer.

Stage III: The cancer has spread to nearby lymph nodes, but not to other parts of the body. Dukes' C is another name for Stage III colorectal cancer.

Stage IV: The cancer has spread to other parts of the body, such as the liver or lungs. Dukes' D is another name for Stage IV colorectal cancer.

Understanding Leukemia

What Is Leukemia?

Leukemia is a cancer of the blood or bone marrow characterized by an abnormal production of white blood cells in the body. The leukemia cells generally look different from normal blood cells and they do not function properly. Over time, leukemic cells may crowd out other types of blood cells, thereby affecting the production of normal red and white blood cells, and platelets.

Blood Cell Development

Blood cells are produced inside the bone in a spongy space called the bone marrow. The process of blood cell formation is called hematopoiesis. All blood cells have a common origin called a stem cell. Stem cells develop into specific mature blood cells by a process called differentiation. Early immature cells are called blasts, which grow into mature blood cells. Once the cells are matured, they are released into the blood where they circulate throughout the body and perform their respective functions.

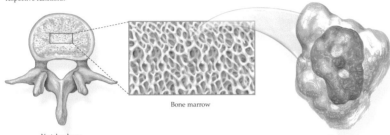

Vertebra bone
Bone marrow
Stem cell

What Is the Function of Blood?

Blood is continuously circulating through the blood vessels carrying vital elements to every part of the body. The blood plays an important role in transporting nutrients from the digestive tract to the body tissues. Oxygen is transported from the lungs to other cells of the body. Waste from cells is carried to the respiratory and excretory organs through the blood. Hormones are transported from the endocrine glands to target tissues via blood. White blood cells participate in the body's immune system to help fight infections and diseases.

What Are the Causes and the Risk Factors?

The exact cause of leukemia is still unknown, but it is influenced by both genetic and environmental factors such as:

- Genetic predisposition
- Environmental exposure to chemicals and/or radiation
- Immunologic factors
- Myelodysplastic syndrome (disease of the blood)

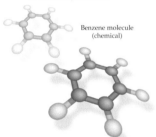

Benzene molecule (chemical)

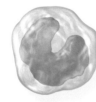

Myelodysplastic syndrome (disease)

Chromosome (genetic)

What Are the Treatment Options?

A person with **acute lymphoblastic leukemia** or **acute myeloid leukemia** needs to be treated right away with chemotherapy (drugs that destroy cancer cells).

Acute Lymphoblastic Leukemia (ALL) – chemotherapy involves multiple phases, which can vary according to protocols.
- Induction phase – large doses of anticancer drugs are used (4-5 drugs given over 1 month).
- Consolidation phase – new combination of drugs are used to destroy any leukemia cells that are still "hiding" within the body.
- Delayed intensification phase – the goal is to give intense chemotherapy when the amount of leukemia cells are low.
- Maintenance phase – used to keep the leukemia in remission (can last 18 months to 2.5 years).
- CNS prophylactic (preventive) therapy – since ALL may spread to the coverings of the brain and spinal cord, medication is given directly into the spinal fluid using a lumbar puncture (spinal tap).

Chronic Lymphocytic Leukemia (CLL) – therapy options include:
- Observation or "watchful waiting" for a patient who has no symptoms, large lymph nodes, and normal red cell and platelet counts.
- Chemotherapy – single or combination of drugs are used.
- Monoclonal antibodies – created in the lab to specifically react with certain types of cancer cells. This can help the patient's immune system to respond and destroy these cancer cells.

Acute Myeloid Leukemia (AML) – chemotherapy involves:
- Induction phase – usually 2 chemotherapy drugs are used and sometimes a third drug is added.
- Consolidation phase – usually involves 2-4 cycles of additional chemotherapy.
- Maintenance phase – not used in AML, except in a variant known as Acute Promyelocytic Leukemia.

Chronic Myeloid Leukemia (CML) – initial therapy involves:
- Imatinib – an oral drug specifically designed to target and interfere with the growth of a protein made by CML cells.

Allogeneic Stem Cell Transplantation (SCT) – is a procedure where healthy bone marrow cells (stem cells) from a donor are transplanted into a leukemia patient. This treatment may be used for all types of leukemia, but it is done only after chemotherapy has been initiated.

Stem Cell Transplant...
- Is seldom used in pediatric ALL, but it is used in adult ALL.
- Is rarely used in CLL patients, since this type of leukemia usually occurs in older patients and the course is often prolonged with multiple therapeutic options.
- Is considered at early stages of AML.
- May still be considered for young CML patients with a matched sibling or for patients who are not responding well to Imatinib.

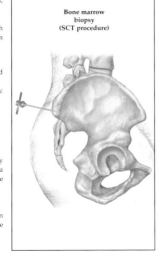

Bone marrow biopsy (SCT procedure)

Types of Leukemia

Leukemias are grouped by how quickly the disease develops and progresses:
- **Acute leukemia** – gets worse quickly as the production of abnormal cells increases rapidly.
- **Chronic leukemia** – gets worse slowly and symptoms may not appear for a long time.

Leukemias are also grouped by the type of white blood cells that are affected.
- When leukemia affects lymphoid cells, it is called **lymphocytic leukemia**.
- When myeloid cells are affected, the disease is called **myeloid** or **myelogenous leukemia**.

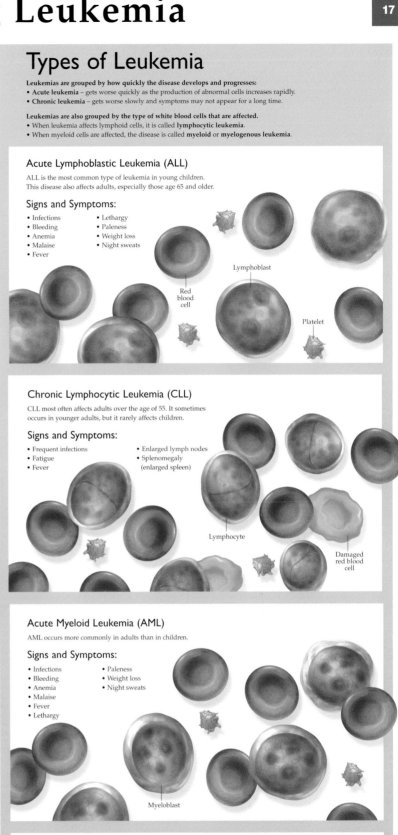

Acute Lymphoblastic Leukemia (ALL)

ALL is the most common type of leukemia in young children. This disease also affects adults, especially those age 65 and older.

Signs and Symptoms:
- Infections
- Bleeding
- Anemia
- Malaise
- Fever
- Lethargy
- Paleness
- Weight loss
- Night sweats

Lymphoblast
Red blood cell
Platelet

Chronic Lymphocytic Leukemia (CLL)

CLL most often affects adults over the age of 55. It sometimes occurs in younger adults, but it rarely affects children.

Signs and Symptoms:
- Frequent infections
- Fatigue
- Fever
- Enlarged lymph nodes
- Splenomegaly (enlarged spleen)

Lymphocyte
Damaged red blood cell

Acute Myeloid Leukemia (AML)

AML occurs more commonly in adults than in children.

Signs and Symptoms:
- Infections
- Bleeding
- Anemia
- Malaise
- Fever
- Lethargy
- Paleness
- Weight loss
- Night sweats

Myeloblast

Chronic Myeloid Leukemia (CML)

CML occurs mainly in adults. Most people with CML are found to have an abnormal chromosome known as the Philadelphia chromosome. This chromosome causes the cell to make a protein which promotes the leukemic cells to grow and multiply.

Signs and Symptoms:
- Heat intolerance
- Splenomegaly (enlarged spleen)
- Weight loss
- Weakness
- Fatigue
- Fever
- Bruising
- Joint pain

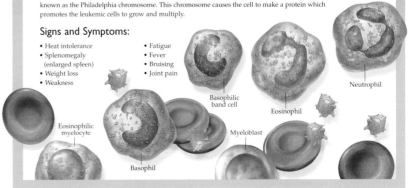

Eosinophilic myelocyte
Basophil
Basophilic band cell
Eosinophil
Myeloblast
Neutrophil

©2008 Wolters Kluwer | Lippincott Williams & Wilkins I Published by **Anatomical Chart Company, Skokie, IL**
Health

Understanding Lung Cancer

Lung cancer is the rapid growth of abnormal (malignant) cells in one or both of the lungs. It can invade nearby tissues and may spread (metastasize) to other areas of the body.

Trachea

Lymph nodes

Metastasis to paratracheal lymph nodes

Bronchus

Tumor projecting into bronchi

Metastasis to carinal lymph nodes

LEFT UPPER LOBE

Tumor projecting into bronchi

LEFT LOWER LOBE

There are 2 Major Types of Lung Cancer: Non-Small Cell Lung Cancer and Small Cell Lung Cancer

Non-small cell lung cancer (NSCLC) is more common than small cell lung cancer, accounting for about 85% of all lung cancers; it generally grows and spreads more slowly. The three most common type of non-small cell lung cancer are:

1. **Adenocarcinoma** are the most common sub-type of NSCLC. It is usually found in the outer part of the lung.
2. **Squamous cell carcinoma** are tumors found near a bronchus.
3. **Large cell carcinoma** is a fast-growing form that can develop in any part of the lung.

NSCLC is staged according to the size of the tumor, the level of lymph node involvement, and the extent to which the cancer has spread. Stages include:

Stage 0   Cancer is limited to the lining of the air passages and has not yet invaded the lung tissue.

Stage I   Cancer has invaded the underlying lung tissue, but has not yet spread to the lymph nodes.

Stage II   Cancer has spread to the neighboring lymph nodes or have spread to the chest wall, or the diaphragm, or the pleura between the lungs, or membranes surrounding the heart.

Stage III   Cancer has spread from the lung to either the lymph nodes in the center of the chest or the collarbone area. The cancer may have spread locally to areas such as the heart, blood, vessels, trachea, and esophagus.

Stage IV   Cancer has spread to other parts of the body, such as the liver, bones, or brain.

Small cell lung cancer (SCLC), also known as oat cell cancer, is the less common form of lung cancer. It is a fast-growing cancer that forms in the tissues of the lungs and spreads to other parts of the body.

SCLC is staged differently from non-small cell types. Rather than using numbers, it is classified as either limited or extensive.

Limited   Cancer is confined to one lung and to its neighboring lymph nodes.

Extensive   Cancer has spread beyond one lung and nearby lymph nodes; it may have invaded both lungs, more remote lymph nodes, or other organs.

How is Lung Cancer Diagnosed?

The tests used to diagnose whether a patient has lung cancer varies depending on the patient's symptoms.

Chest X-Ray – Most patients under go this test to see if there are any abnormalities.

Chest CT Scan – If an abnormality is discovered in the chest x-ray, a computerized tomography (CT) scan is performed to provide a series of detailed pictures of parts inside the body, taken from different angles.

Biopsy – There are several different types of biopsy procedures. The choice of procedure, which may involve surgery, will depend on what is discovered via the chest x-ray and/or chest CT scan.

Sputum Cytology – A sample of phlegm is examined under a microscope.

CHEST X-RAY   CT SCAN   PET SCAN   MRI

How is Lung Cancer Staged?

If cancer is diagnosed, more tests are done so the doctor can plan a treatment. These tests help discover the stage (extent) of the cancer. Common tests include:

Positron Emission Tomography (PET) scan – After a small amount of radioactive glucose (sugar) is injected into a vein of a patient, a special camera makes computerized pictures highlighting potential cancer cells.

PET/CT Scan – PET scan information is combined with the anatomical information from a CT scan to reliably determine whether an abnormal growth is cancerous or benign (non-cancerous).

Magnetic Resonance Imaging (MRI) of the Head – A powerful magnet linked to a computer produces detailed images of the areas inside the head.

Mediastinoscopy/Mediastinotomy – A lighted instrument (scope) is inserted into the body to examine the chest and nearby lymph nodes.

Risk Factors

- **Smoking cigarettes, cigars, and pipes**
- **Exposure to:**
  - **Secondhand smoke**
  - **Radon** – Radioactive gas that occurs naturally in soil and rocks. Mine workers may be exposed to radon. Radon may also be found in homes and buildings
  - **Asbestos** – Group of naturally-occurring fibrous minerals that are used in certain industries.
  - **Pollution**
- **Having previous lung diseases, such as tuberculosis (TB) and emphysema**
- **Personal history** – A person with a history of lung cancer is more likely to develop it again than someone who has never had the disease.
- **Heredity** – Genetics seem to play a role in who develops lung cancer

Signs and Symptoms

- **Cough that does not go away**
- **Constant chest pain**
- **Coughing up blood**
- **Shortness of breath, wheezing, or hoarseness**
- **Problems with pneumonia or bronchitis**
- **Swelling of the neck and face**
- **Loss of appetite and/or weight**
- **Fatigue**

If lung cancer has spread to other organs (metastasized), signs may include headaches, visual changes, stroke-like symptoms (if cancer has spread to the brain), and bone pain (if the cancer has spread to the bones).

Treatment Options

Treatment depends on a number of factors including the type of lung cancer, the size/location/stage of the tumor, and the general health and pulmonary function of the patient. Many different types of treatments or combination of treatments may be used, such as:

Surgical Resection – A portion of the lung containing the tumor is removed. Depending on the case, the surgeon may remove only a small portion, the entire lobe (lobectomy), or the entire lung (pneumonectomy). Lymph nodes are also sampled at the time of surgery. Lobectomy is the most widely used surgical procedure for lung cancer.

Chemotherapy – The use of anticancer drugs that kill cancer cells throughout the body.

Radiation therapy – The use of high-energy rays to kill cancer cells. This therapy is directed to a limited area and affects the cancer cells only in that area.

Endobronchial Therapy – A group of therapies used to treat lesions that are accessible in the lung airways. They are primarily used for palliative therapy (to relieve symptoms, not to cure the disease), but may also be used for early stages of the disease.

How can Lung Cancer be Prevented?

- **Don't smoke** – If you do smoke, quit. If you stop smoking, the risk of lung cancer decreases each year as normal cells replace abnormal cells. After 10 years, the risk drops to a level that is one-third to one-half of the risk of people who continue to smoke.
- **Avoid secondhand smoke**
- **Test your home for radon**
- **Avoid carcinogens** - People who are exposed to large amounts of asbestos should use protective equipment.

APPROXIMATELY 90% OF LUNG CANCER DEATHS ARE RELATED TO SMOKING

Understanding Skin Cancer

What Causes Skin Cancer?

Skin cancer is the uncontrolled growth of abnormal cells in a layer of the skin. It attacks one out of seven Americans each year. The total amount of sun exposure received over many years and single overexposures resulting in sunburn both can cause skin cancer.

Noon

3:00PM

9:00AM

Due to the changing angle of our sun and the absorption of solar radiation by our atmosphere, the intensity of ultraviolet radiation striking the surface of the earth at noon is twice as strong as radiation striking the earth in the early morning and late afternoon.

UVA and UVB absorption by DNA and other structures inside the nuclei of skin cells leads to cellular and molecular damage (sunburn), including pain, inflammation, swelling, and loss of function.

Keratinocyte (can become squamous cell carcinoma)

Nucleus

DNA

Cell nucleus

Arteriole

Basal cell (can become basal cell carcinoma)

Incomplete or incorrect repair of ultraviolet radiation-induced DNA damage is largely responsible for the growth of precancerous cells and malignant cells.

1. Golgi apparatus (produces melanosomes)

2. Melanosomes (develop into granules)

3. Melanin granules (store melanin pigment for transport to keratinocytes)

Melanocyte (can become melanoma)

Melanocytes located in the basal layer of the epidermis produce melanin, a pigment that is responsible for the various skin colors.

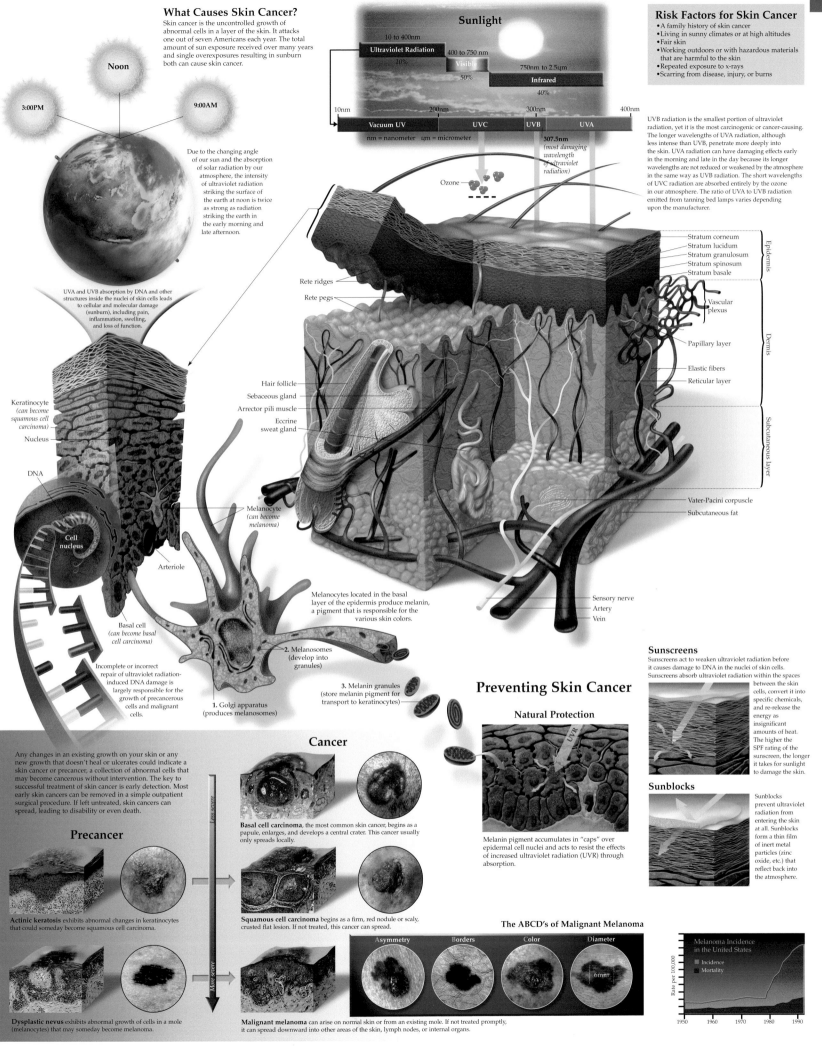

Sunlight

10 to 400nm

Ultraviolet Radiation 10%

400 to 750 nm
Visible 50%

750nm to 2.5μm
Infrared 40%

10nm   200nm   300nm   400nm

| Vacuum UV | UVC | UVB | UVA |

nm = nanometer   μm = micrometer

307.5nm (most damaging wavelength of ultraviolet radiation)

Ozone

UVB radiation is the smallest portion of ultraviolet radiation, yet it is the most carcinogenic or cancer-causing. The longer wavelengths of UVA radiation, although less intense than UVB, penetrate more deeply into the skin. UVA radiation can have damaging effects early in the morning and late in the day because its longer wavelengths are not reduced or weakened by the atmosphere in the same way as UVB radiation. The short wavelengths of UVC radiation are absorbed entirely by the ozone in our atmosphere. The ratio of UVA to UVB radiation emitted from tanning bed lamps varies depending upon the manufacturer.

Rete ridges

Rete pegs

Hair follicle
Sebaceous gland
Arrector pili muscle
Eccrine sweat gland

Stratum corneum
Stratum lucidum
Stratum granulosum
Stratum spinosum
Stratum basale

Epidermis

Vascular plexus

Papillary layer

Elastic fibers
Reticular layer

Dermis

Subcutaneous layer

Vater-Pacini corpuscle
Subcutaneous fat

Sensory nerve
Artery
Vein

Risk Factors for Skin Cancer

- A family history of skin cancer
- Living in sunny climates or at high altitudes
- Fair skin
- Working outdoors or with hazardous materials that are harmful to the skin
- Repeated exposure to x-rays
- Scarring from disease, injury, or burns

Preventing Skin Cancer

Natural Protection

Melanin pigment accumulates in "caps" over epidermal cell nuclei and acts to resist the effects of increased ultraviolet radiation (UVR) through absorption.

Sunscreens

Sunscreens act to weaken ultraviolet radiation before it causes damage to DNA in the nuclei of skin cells. Sunscreens absorb ultraviolet radiation within the spaces between the skin cells, convert it into specific chemicals, and re-release the energy as insignificant amounts of heat. The higher the SPF rating of the sunscreen, the longer it takes for sunlight to damage the skin.

Sunblocks

Sunblocks prevent ultraviolet radiation from entering the skin at all. Sunblocks form a thin film of inert metal particles (zinc oxide, etc.) that reflect back into the atmosphere.

Cancer

Any changes in an existing growth on your skin or any new growth that doesn't heal or ulcerates could indicate a skin cancer or precancer, a collection of abnormal cells that may become cancerous without intervention. The key to successful treatment of skin cancer is early detection. Most early skin cancers can be removed in a simple outpatient surgical procedure. If left untreated, skin cancers can spread, leading to disability or even death.

Less severe / More severe

Basal cell carcinoma, the most common skin cancer, begins as a papule, enlarges, and develops a central crater. This cancer usually only spreads locally.

Squamous cell carcinoma begins as a firm, red nodule or scaly, crusted flat lesion. If not treated, this cancer can spread.

Precancer

Actinic keratosis exhibits abnormal changes in keratinocytes that could someday become squamous cell carcinoma.

Dysplastic nevus exhibits abnormal growth of cells in a mole (melanocytes) that may someday become melanoma.

The ABCD's of Malignant Melanoma

Asymmetry   **Borders**   **Color**   **Diameter**

6mm

Malignant melanoma can arise on normal skin or from an existing mole. If not treated promptly, it can spread downward into other areas of the skin, lymph nodes, or internal organs.

Melanoma Incidence in the United States

Incidence
Mortality

Rate per 100,000

1950   1960   1970   1980   1990

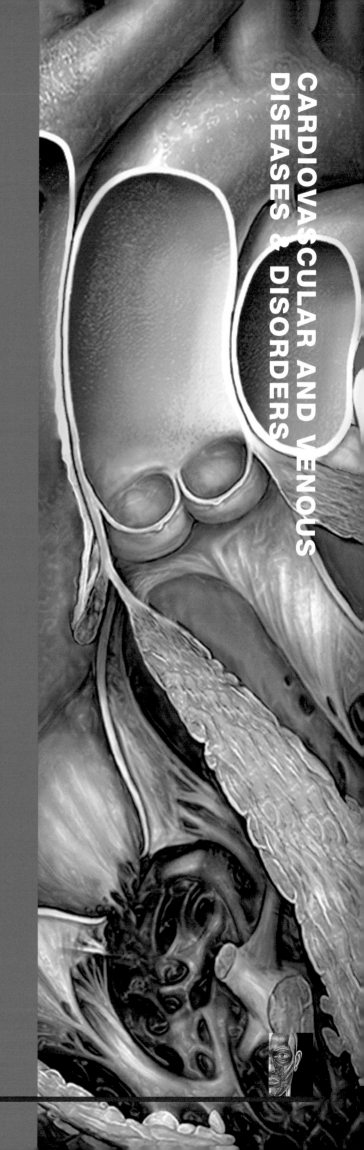

CARDIOVASCULAR AND VENOUS DISEASES & DISORDERS

• Cardiovascular Disease • High Cholesterol • Deep Vein Thrombosis • Heart Conditions • Heart Disease • Understanding Hypertension

Cardiovascular Disease

NORMAL HEART ANATOMY

Cross Section

- Superior vena cava
- Aorta
- Pulmonary trunk
- Right atrium
- Left auricle
- Pulmonary valve
- Mitral valve
- Tricuspid valve
- Left ventricle
- Right ventricle
- Inferior vena cava

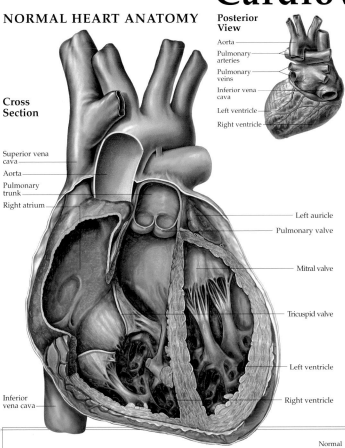

Posterior View

- Aorta
- Pulmonary arteries
- Pulmonary veins
- Inferior vena cava
- Left ventricle
- Right ventricle

Anterior View

- Superior vena cava
- Aorta
- Right atrium
- Pulmonary trunk
- Left auricle
- Right ventricle
- Left ventricle
- Inferior vena cava

Conduction System

- Sinuatrial (S-A) node
- Atrioventricular (A-V) node
- Atrioventricular bundle (Bundle of His)
- Right crus
- Left crus
- Purkinje's fiber

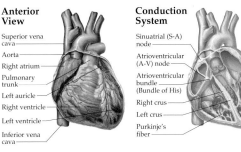

Coronary Arteries (Anterior view)

Coronary arteries supply blood to heart tissue. They originate from the aorta.

- Aorta
- Sinuatrial nodal a.
- R. coronary a.
- R. atrial aa.
- Conus arteriosus br.
- R. anterior ventricular a.
- R. marginal a.
- Posterior descending a.
- L. coronary a.
- Circumflex a.
- Posterior atrial a.
- L. marginal a.
- Diagonal a.
- Left anterior descending a.

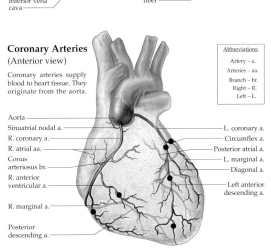

Abbreviations:
Artery – a.
Arteries – aa.
Branch – br.
Right – R.
Left – L.

● *Common areas of coronary artery blockage that result in damage to heart muscle.*

Electrocardiogram (ECG)

Repeating electrical impulses travel through the heart, controlling the rhythmic contraction and dilation of the heart muscle. The impulse is displayed in a waveform with three distinct waves: P, QRS, and T.

The Cardiac Cycle

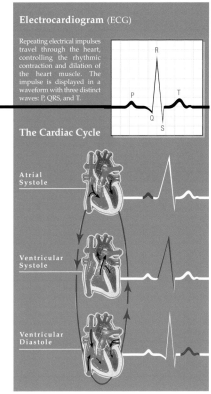

- Atrial Systole
- Ventricular Systole
- Ventricular Diastole

CARDIOVASCULAR DISEASE

Polyarteritis Nodosa (PAN)

Aneurysm

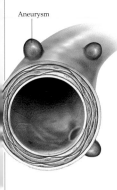

Polyarteritis nodosa (PAN) is a disease of inflammation of the small and medium-sized blood vessels, which can involve multiple organs of the body. The organs most commonly involved are the kidneys, heart, liver, and gastrointestinal tract. Less commonly involved are the muscles, brain, spinal cord, peripheral nerves, and skin. The inflammation can cause beadlike aneurysms of the involved blood vessels, which cause decreased blood flow to the affected organs.

Kawasaki's Disease

Inflammation of blood vessel

Also known as mucocutaneous lymph node syndrome, Kawasaki's disease is a multi-organ illness affecting children. It generally starts with high fever, followed by the development of redness and swelling of the hands, feet, eyes, lips, and tongue; swollen lymph glands; and sores in the mouth. Acute complications involving the heart include inflammation of the heart muscle and accumulation of fluid around the heart. Fatal heart attacks occur due to inflammation of the blood vessels (coronary arteries) of the heart, causing blood clots to form and block the arteries. Chronic complications include aneurysms of the coronary arteries that can rupture in adulthood.

Cerebrovascular Accident (Stroke)

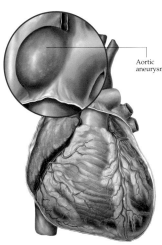

Blood clot

A cerebrovascular accident (CVA), also known as a stroke, is a sudden impairment of cerebral circulation in one or more blood vessels. This interrupts or diminishes oxygen supply to the brain, often causing the brain tissues to become damaged or die.

Coronary Artery Disease

Normal Coronary Artery — Fatty Streak

Fibrous Plaque — Complicated Plaque

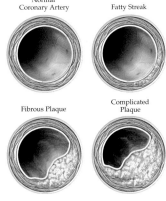

If excessive amounts of fat are circulating in the blood, the arteries can accumulate fatty deposits called plaques. This buildup, called atherosclerosis, causes the vessels to narrow or become obstructed. Coronary artery disease results as atherosclerotic plaque fills the lumens of the coronary arteries and obstructs blood flow to the heart. This results in diminished supply of oxygen and nutrients to the heart tissue.

Aortic Aneurysm

Aortic aneurysm

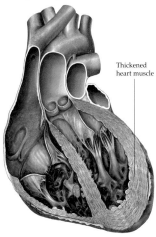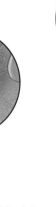

The aorta is the largest blood vessel in the body. It comes out of the top of the heart and brings blood to the rest of the body. Atherosclerosis can cause the wall of the aorta to weaken and balloon out (aneurysm). The aortic aneurysm may suddenly rupture or tear, often leading to death.

Angina

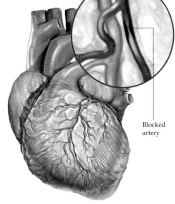

Blocked artery

The coronary arteries supplying the heart can become narrowed over time, due to age, hereditary factors, chronic smoking, high cholesterol, high blood pressure, or diabetes. The narrowed blood vessels limit the amount of blood flow to the heart, especially with strenuous activity. When the heart muscle is not getting enough blood, pain or discomfort in the chest, commonly called angina, results.

Left Ventricular Hypertrophy (LVH)

Thickened heart muscle

LVH is when the muscle of the heart's left ventricle becomes thickened and enlarged. The heart then becomes less efficient at circulating blood throughout the body. The resulting condition is called congestive heart failure. This may cause the lungs to fill up with fluid, resulting in difficulty breathing, fluid retention and swollen legs, and decreased blood flow to various parts of the body.

Myocardial Infarction (Heart Attack)

Infarction

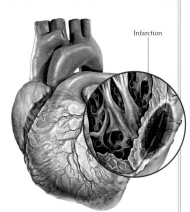

Myocardial infarction occurs when a coronary artery narrowed by atherosclerosis becomes completely blocked. This is usually the result of a blood clot that forms where the artery is narrowed. The blocked artery prevents the heart from receiving oxygen, and part or all of the heart muscle is either damaged (infarction) or dies. The damaged part of the heart loses its ability to contract and pump blood to and from the heart.

Congestive Heart Failure

Dilated ventricle

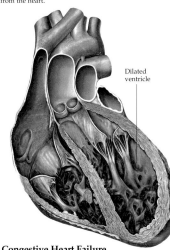

Congestive heart failure is a common debilitating condition defined by the heart's mechanical inability to pump blood effectively. The result is a decrease in blood circulation, which forces blood to back up and oxygen supply to decrease in muscle and lung tissues. Excess accumulation of fluids in tissues throughout the body causes swelling (edema), which impairs the function of affected organs.

High Cholesterol

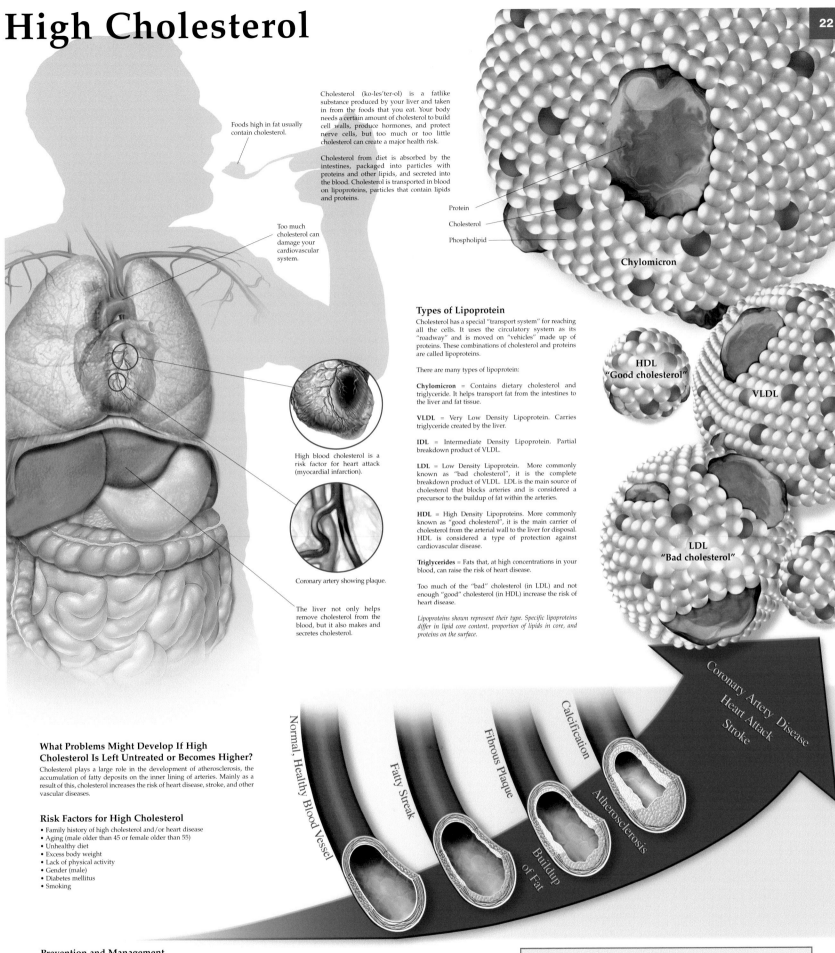

Foods high in fat usually contain cholesterol.

Cholesterol (ko-les'ter-ol) is a fatlike substance produced by your liver and taken in from the foods that you eat. Your body needs a certain amount of cholesterol to build cell walls, produce hormones, and protect nerve cells, but too much or too little cholesterol can create a major health risk.

Cholesterol from diet is absorbed by the intestines, packaged into particles with proteins and other lipids, and secreted into the blood. Cholesterol is transported in blood on lipoproteins, particles that contain lipids and proteins.

Too much cholesterol can damage your cardiovascular system.

Protein
Cholesterol
Phospholipid

Chylomicron

HDL
"Good cholesterol"

VLDL

LDL
"Bad cholesterol"

High blood cholesterol is a risk factor for heart attack (myocardial infarction).

Coronary artery showing plaque.

The liver not only helps remove cholesterol from the blood, but it also makes and secretes cholesterol.

Types of Lipoprotein

Cholesterol has a special "transport system" for reaching all the cells. It uses the circulatory system as its "roadway" and is moved on "vehicles" made up of proteins. These combinations of cholesterol and proteins are called lipoproteins.

There are many types of lipoprotein:

Chylomicron = Contains dietary cholesterol and triglyceride. It helps transport fat from the intestines to the liver and fat tissue.

VLDL = Very Low Density Lipoprotein. Carries triglyceride created by the liver.

IDL = Intermediate Density Lipoprotein. Partial breakdown product of VLDL.

LDL = Low Density Lipoprotein. More commonly known as "bad cholesterol", it is the complete breakdown product of VLDL. LDL is the main source of cholesterol that blocks arteries and is considered a precursor to the buildup of fat within the arteries.

HDL = High Density Lipoproteins. More commonly known as "good cholesterol", it is the main carrier of cholesterol from the arterial wall to the liver for disposal. HDL is considered a type of protection against cardiovascular disease.

Triglycerides = Fats that, at high concentrations in your blood, can raise the risk of heart disease.

Too much of the "bad" cholesterol (in LDL) and not enough "good" cholesterol (in HDL) increase the risk of heart disease.

Lipoproteins shown represent their type. Specific lipoproteins differ in lipid core content, proportion of lipids in core, and proteins on the surface.

Normal, Healthy Blood Vessel
Fatty Streak
Fibrous Plaque
Calcification
Atherosclerosis
Buildup of Fat
Coronary Artery Disease
Heart Attack
Stroke

What Problems Might Develop If High Cholesterol Is Left Untreated or Becomes Higher?

Cholesterol plays a large role in the development of atherosclerosis, the accumulation of fatty deposits on the inner lining of arteries. Mainly as a result of this, cholesterol increases the risk of heart disease, stroke, and other vascular diseases.

Risk Factors for High Cholesterol

- Family history of high cholesterol and/or heart disease
- Aging (male older than 45 or female older than 55)
- Unhealthy diet
- Excess body weight
- Lack of physical activity
- Gender (male)
- Diabetes mellitus
- Smoking

Prevention and Management

1. Get regular cholesterol screenings: The first step in preventing high cholesterol and ultimately, coronary artery disease, is to get a simple blood test to check your cholesterol levels. Getting the complete lipid profile test is helpful in understanding your cholesterol levels. Healthy adults should have this test done every five years. If you are at increased risk for heart disease or if you are a man over 45 or a woman over 55, your doctor might have you tested more often.

2. Adopt a healthier lifestyle: Engaging in regular aerobic exercise, quitting smoking, maintaining a healthy weight, and eating a low-fat diet can reduce your risk of developing high cholesterol. Even those with a low blood cholesterol level should still eat a diet low in saturated fat and cholesterol, and should adopt and maintain a physically active lifestyle.

3. Lower LDL levels:
Clinical trials have demonstrated that lowering LDL cholesterol has many benefits and saves lives. The benefits include:
- Preventing plaque rupture
- Decreasing the risk of heart attack
- Lowering the risk of stroke
- Reducing the formation of new cholesterol plaques
- Reducing the burden of existing plaques

The HDL cholesterol level is thought to be important in preventing heart disease. Lower HDL cholesterol levels are strongly associated with increased risk of heart disease. Therefore, an HDL cholesterol level above 40 mg/dL or 1 mmol/L is more beneficial.

4. Take cholesterol medications, if prescribed by a health practicioner: Even after adopting a healthier lifestyle, your cholesterol level may not reach target and a medication may be required.

Desirable Cholesterol Levels*

Target Total Cholesterol Level
Under 200 mg/dL (Under 5 mmol/L)

Target LDL Level
Under 100 mg/dL (Under 3 mmol/L)

*These levels should be used as a general guideline. Current recommendations might have changed and should be followed instead of what is stated here. Target levels also differ according to the number of risk factors you have for coronary artery disease. Please see your doctor to find out what your target level should be.

©2008 ● Wolters Kluwer | Lippincott Williams & Wilkins | Published by Anatomical Chart Company, Skokie, IL
Health

Deep Vein Thrombosis

Vascular Circulation

The circulation of blood through the blood vessels *(arteries, capillaries, and veins)* of the body is driven by the beating action of the heart. The heart beats at a rate of about 70 beats per minute, forcing blood into the arteries, which in turn transports oxygen and nutrients throughout the body. After exchanging oxygen for carbon dioxide and nutrients for waste products, the blood begins its journey back to the heart through a network of veins. On returning to the heart, the non-oxygenated blood is pumped into the arteries of the lungs *(pulmonary arteries)*, where the blood regains oxygen. Then the blood re-enters the heart through the pulmonary veins for another cycle. The entire cycle takes about a minute to complete.

Enlarged view of lung

Pulmonary arterial circulation shown in blue *(non-oxygenated blood)*

Pulmonary venous circulation shown in red *(oxygenated blood)*

Embolus

Pulmonary artery

Pulmonary Embolism

A pulmonary embolus is a piece of blood clot *(venous thrombus)* that has broken off and traveled into a pulmonary artery of the lungs. If the embolus is very large, it can block blood flow into the pulmonary arteries. This is called pulmonary embolism. This causes severe breathing difficulties and can even cause death. Smaller pulmonary emboli can cause chest pain or cause no symptoms. With time, the smaller emboli are either dissolved or break up and disappear.

External iliac vein

Femoral vein

Tunica intima

Tunica media

Tunica adventitia

Thrombus *(blood clot)* blocking blood flow through a vein

Posterior tibial vein

Perineal vein

Cross-Section of a Vein

○ The circles show locations in the veins commonly affected by deep vein thrombosis *(applies to both legs)*.

↑ The arrows show the direction of the venous blood flow back to the heart and then into the lungs.

Lung

Pulmonary artery

Heart

Abdominal aorta

Inferior vena cava

Common iliac vein

Common iliac artery

Femoral artery

Embolus *(a broken-off piece of thrombus)*

Venous thrombus *(blood clot)*

Direction of blood flow

Clumping of:
Fibrin
Platelet
Red blood cell

Ⓐ Damage to the inner lining of blood vessel

How Does a Thrombus (*Blood Clot*) Form?

1. Under normal circumstances blood remains fluid because the lining *(endothelium)* of blood vessels contains substances that prevent it from clotting.

2. Blood clotting is important because it prevents excessive blood loss when a vessel is cut. Ⓐ There are substances in the inner layer of a blood vessel that stimulate blood clotting *(coagulation)*. Ⓑ A clot forms when blood is exposed to these substances.

3. Under certain abnormal circumstances, the blood can clot to produce a thrombus, Ⓒ even though the blood vessel is not cut. These abnormal circumstances cause clotting either by releasing chemicals into the blood or cause damage to the inner lining of the vessel, thereby removing the inner protective layer.

4. The chance of clotting is increased if the blood flow is sluggish *(stagnant)*. Blood flow can become sluggish because of prolonged bed rest or when there is an inherited defect in the body's ability to counteract a tendency to clot.

5. A venous thrombus is made up of a fibrin mesh with trapped blood cells. The thrombus can block the vein, grow, be dissolved by the body– or a piece of it can break off. The broken-off piece *(embolus)* can travel to the lungs, where it is called a pulmonary embolus. Ⓓ

Layers That Makes Up a Vein

Tunica adventitia

External elastic membrane

Tunica media

Internal elastic membrane

Tunica intima *(endothelium)*

Valve

What Is Deep Vein Thrombosis?

Deep vein thrombosis (DVT), or venous thrombosis, occurs when a blood clot forms in the deep veins of the legs. It usually starts in the calf veins and may extend into the thigh veins. A blood clot is a jelly-like mass of congealed blood.

What Causes Deep Vein Thrombosis?

Deep vein thrombosis occurs when blood, which is normally fluid, is stimulated to clot. This happens because the vessel is damaged or substances that trigger blood clotting *(coagulation)* are released into the blood by inflamed or damaged tissues. Blood clotting is encouraged by sluggish blood flow *(venous stasis)*.

What Are the Consequences of DVT?

If the blood clot is small, it can be dissolved by the body. On the other hand, it can grow and block the blood flow through the vein. This causes pain and leg swelling. If a piece of the blood clot *(thrombus)* breaks off, it is called an embolus. A pulmonary embolus is a piece of blood clot that has traveled to the lungs.

What Are the Main Risk Factors?

The risk factors for venous thrombosis are:
- Prolonged bed rest.
- Long periods of immobility *(such as traveling on a long airplane flight)*.
- Varicose veins.
- Major surgery.
- Leg trauma.
- The hormone estrogen in contraceptive pills or hormone replacement therapy.
- Previous venous thrombosis.
- Hereditary predisposition because of abnormal anticoagulant proteins.
- Cancer *(malignancy)*.
- Overweight *(obesity)*.

What Are the Symptoms and Complications of DVT and Pulmonary Embolism?

Many venous thrombi cause no symptoms. The common symptoms are:
- Pain, tenderness and/or swelling in the calf or elsewhere in the leg.
- Discoloration of the calf.
- Symptoms of pulmonary embolism.

The symptoms of pulmonary embolism are:
- Difficulty in breathing.
- Sharp chest pain that is aggravated by taking a deep breath.
- Blood in sputum.
- Rapid heart rate.

The complications of DVT are **(1)** chronic pain and swelling of the leg because of scarring of the valves within the vein and blockage of blood flow, and **(2)** pulmonary embolism, which occurs when a blood clot fragment, which has broken off from a venous thrombus, enters and blocks a pulmonary artery. A very large embolus can block blood flow into the pulmonary arteries and cause death. Smaller pulmonary emboli obstruct smaller arteries and can cause damage to the lungs. Many pulmonary emboli do not cause symptoms. With time, most pulmonary emboli are dissolved by the body.

How Are DVT and Pulmonary Embolism Treated?

Treatment of deep vein thrombosis is aimed at relieving symptoms, preventing the blood clot from growing and preventing pulmonary embolism.

This is achieved by:
- Blood-thinning drugs known as anticoagulants.
- In cases of large pulmonary embolism, clot dissolving drugs.
- Compression stocking to counteract swelling in the leg, if it is still present after three months.
- Surgery can be used to prevent a venous thrombus from traveling to the lungs, but this is rarely necessary.

Heart Conditions

Heart Murmurs

A heart murmur is an extra or abnormal sound produced by the heart, which can be heard with a stethoscope. A common cause of heart murmur is turbulent blood flow. This can be due to:

- Holes in the heart walls (ventricular septal defect, atrial septal defect).
- Defective heart valves (mitral valve prolapse, pulmonary valve stenosis, aortic stenosis).
- Abnormalities of the heart chambers (infundibular stenosis).
- Narrowing of a major artery (coarctation of the aorta).

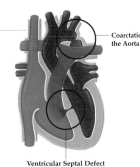

Coarctation of the Aorta

Ventricular Septal Defect

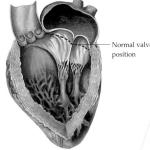

Normal valve position

Mitral Valve Prolapse

Normal Anatomy of the Heart

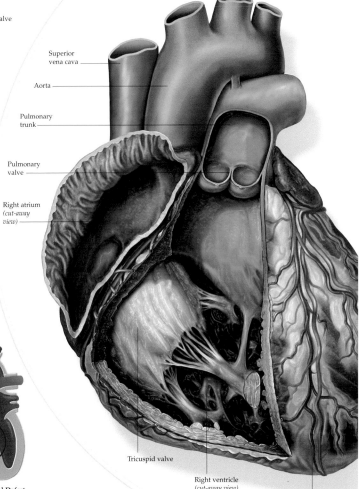

- Superior vena cava
- Aorta
- Pulmonary trunk
- Pulmonary valve
- Right atrium (cut-away view)
- Tricuspid valve
- Right ventricle (cut-away view)
- Left ventricle

Cardiac Arrhythmias

In cardiac arrhythmias, abnormal electrical conduction changes the heart rate and rhythm. Common arrhythmias include:

- **Tachycardia** is a rapid heartbeat (more than 100 beats/min.) that can cause inefficient blood circulation. Symptoms include palpitations (rapid throbbing of the heart), dizziness, lightheadedness, and fainting.
- **Bradycardia** is a slowed heartbeat (less than 60 beats/min.) that causes a person to feel fatigued, dizzy, lightheaded, and may trigger fainting.
- **Atrial fibrillation** develops when a disturbance in the electrical signals causes the two atrial chambers of the heart to quiver rather than pump correctly.
- **Ventricular arrhythmias** are the most severe and life threatening. They affect the ventricles, which are the main pumping chambers of the heart.

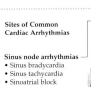

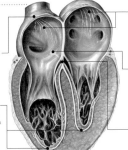

Sites of Common Cardiac Arrhythmias

Sinus node arrhythmias
- Sinus bradycardia
- Sinus tachycardia
- Sinoatrial block

Ventricular arrhythmias
- Ventricular fibrillation
- Ventricular tachycardia
- Premature ventricular contractions

Atrial arrhythmias
- Atrial fibrillation
- Atrial flutter
- Premature atrial contractions

Atrioventricular (AV) blocks
- 1st-degree AV block
- 2nd-degree AV block
- 3rd-degree AV block

Junctional arrhythmias
- AV junctional rhythm

Congenital Heart Defects

Congenital heart defects are problems with the heart's structure that are present at birth. These structural problems can affect the proper function of the heart. The most common heart defects includes patent ductus arteriosus, atrial septal defect, and ventricular septal defect.

- **Patent ductus arteriosus** – the lumen of the duct between the aorta and pulmonary artery remains open after birth.
- **Atrial septal defect** – an opening between the left and right atria permits blood flow from left atrium to right atrium rather than from left to left ventricle.
- **Ventricular septal defect** – an opening in the septum between the ventricles that allows blood flow to shunt between the left and right ventricles.

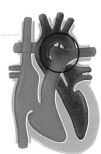
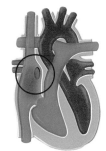
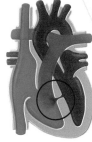

Patent Ductus Arteriosus

Atrial Septal Defect

Ventricular Septal Defect

Acquired Heart Defects

Acquired heart defects are heart problems that develop later in life because of an illness.

- **Myocarditis** – the heart muscle (myocardium) becomes inflamed and may be damaged by a viral infection. The heart muscle weakens and its ability to contract is reduced.
- **Rheumatic heart disease** – caused by rheumatic fever and leads to heart muscle and heart valve damage.
- **Cardiomyopathy** – a disease of the heart muscle caused by a genetic disorder or occurring after an infection.
- **Kawasaki's disease** – an illness that occurs in young children that may leave the heart muscle or coronary arteries damaged.

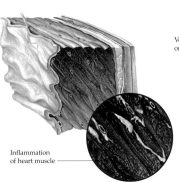

Inflammation of heart muscle

Myocarditis

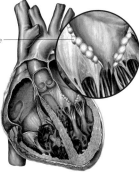

Vegetations on heart valve

Rheumatic Heart Disease

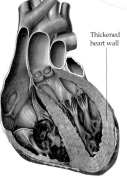

Thickened heart wall

Cardiomyopathy

Inflammation of blood vessel

Kawasaki's Disease

High Cholesterol

Two types of cholesterol are important in heart disease. The first is low-density lipoprotein (LDL) or "bad" cholesterol, which contributes to the buildup of cholesterol in the arteries and to atherosclerosis. The second is high-density lipoprotein (HDL) or "good" cholesterol, which helps keep the "bad" cholesterol from building up in the arteries, thereby lowering heart disease risk.

Coronary Artery Disease (CAD)

If excessive amounts of fat (cholesterol) are circulating in the blood, the arteries can accumulate fatty deposits called plaques. This buildup, called atherosclerosis, causes the vessels to narrow or become obstructed. Coronary artery disease results as atherosclerotic plaque fills the lumens of the coronary arteries and obstructs blood flow to the heart. This results in diminished supply of oxygen and nutrients to the heart tissue. One possible result is myocardial infarction, or heart attack.

Hypertension (high blood pressure)

Hypertension is a major cause of heart disease, stroke, and kidney failure. When blood pressure is elevated, the heart must work harder to pump blood through the arteries. Over time, this can cause thickening of the heart muscle and hardening of the arteries (arteriosclerosis). Eventually, the heart muscle may not get enough blood flow and may not be able to function properly.

Other conditions that can affect the heart include diabetes and overweight/obesity.

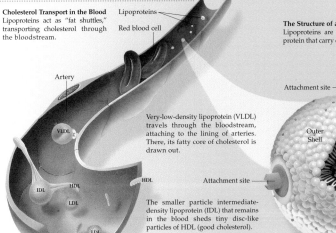
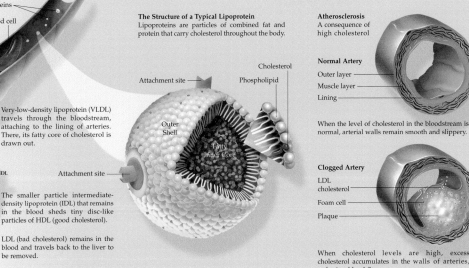

Cholesterol Transport in the Blood
Lipoproteins act as "fat shuttles," transporting cholesterol through the bloodstream.

Lipoproteins

Red blood cell

Artery

VLDL

IDL

HDL

LDL

Very-low-density lipoprotein (VLDL) travels through the bloodstream, attaching to the lining of arteries. There, its fatty core of cholesterol is drawn out.

The smaller particle intermediate-density lipoprotein (IDL) that remains in the blood sheds tiny disc-like particles of HDL (good cholesterol).

LDL (bad cholesterol) remains in the blood and travels back to the liver to be removed.

The Structure of a Typical Lipoprotein
Lipoproteins are particles of combined fat and protein that carry cholesterol throughout the body.

Attachment site

Cholesterol

Phospholipid

Outer Shell

Fatty Inner Core

Attachment site

Atherosclerosis
A consequence of high cholesterol

Normal Artery
- Outer layer
- Muscle layer
- Lining

When the level of cholesterol in the bloodstream is normal, arterial walls remain smooth and slippery.

Clogged Artery
- LDL cholesterol
- Foam cell
- Plaque

When cholesterol levels are high, excess cholesterol accumulates in the walls of arteries, reducing blood flow.

©2008 Wolters Kluwer Health | Lippincott Williams & Wilkins I Published by Anatomical Chart Company, Skokie, IL

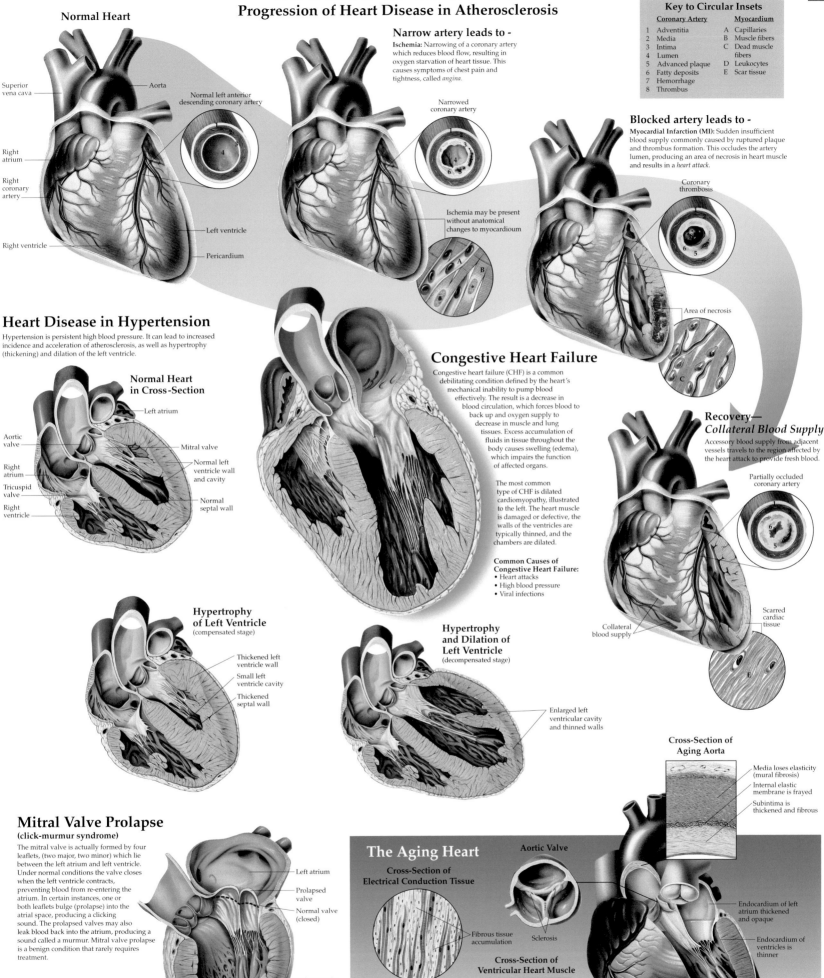

Heart Disease
Progression of Heart Disease in Atherosclerosis

Key to Circular Insets

Coronary Artery	Myocardium
1 Adventitia	A Capillaries
2 Media	B Muscle fibers
3 Intima	C Dead muscle fibers
4 Lumen	D Leukocytes
5 Advanced plaque	E Scar tissue
6 Fatty deposits	
7 Hemorrhage	
8 Thrombus	

Normal Heart

Superior vena cava
Aorta
Normal left anterior descending coronary artery
Right atrium
Right coronary artery
Right ventricle
Left ventricle
Pericardium

Narrow artery leads to -

Ischemia: Narrowing of a coronary artery which reduces blood flow, resulting in oxygen starvation of heart tissue. This causes symptoms of chest pain and tightness, called *angina.*

Narrowed coronary artery

Ischemia may be present without anatomical changes to myocardioum

Blocked artery leads to -

Myocardial Infarction (MI): Sudden insufficient blood supply commonly caused by ruptured plaque and thrombus formation. This occludes the artery lumen, producing an area of necrosis in heart muscle and results in a *heart attack.*

Coronary thrombosis

Area of necrosis

Heart Disease in Hypertension

Hypertension is persistent high blood pressure. It can lead to increased incidence and acceleration of atherosclerosis, as well as hypertrophy (thickening) and dilation of the left ventricle.

Normal Heart in Cross-Section

Left atrium
Aortic valve
Mitral valve
Right atrium
Tricuspid valve
Right ventricle
Normal left ventricle wall and cavity
Normal septal wall

Hypertrophy of Left Ventricle
(compensated stage)

Thickened left ventricle wall
Small left ventricle cavity
Thickened septal wall

Hypertrophy and Dilation of Left Ventricle
(decompensated stage)

Enlarged left ventricular cavity and thinned walls

Congestive Heart Failure

Congestive heart failure (CHF) is a common debilitating condition defined by the heart's mechanical inability to pump blood effectively. The result is a decrease in blood circulation, which forces blood to back up and oxygen supply to decrease in muscle and lung tissues. Excess accumulation of fluids in tissue throughout the body causes swelling (edema), which impairs the function of affected organs.

The most common type of CHF is dilated cardiomyopathy, illustrated to the left. The heart muscle is damaged or defective, the walls of the ventricles are typically thinned, and the chambers are dilated.

Common Causes of Congestive Heart Failure:
• Heart attacks
• High blood pressure
• Viral infections

Recovery—
Collateral Blood Supply

Accessory blood supply from adjacent vessels travels to the region affected by the heart attack to provide fresh blood.

Partially occluded coronary artery
Collateral blood supply
Scarred cardiac tissue

Cross-Section of Aging Aorta

Media loses elasticity (mural fibrosis)
Internal elastic membrane is frayed
Subintima is thickened and fibrous

Mitral Valve Prolapse
(click-murmur syndrome)

The mitral valve is actually formed by four leaflets, (two major, two minor) which lie between the left atrium and left ventricle. Under normal conditions the valve closes when the left ventricle contracts, preventing blood from re-entering the atrium. In certain instances, one or both leaflets bulge (prolapse) into the atrial space, producing a clicking sound. The prolapsed valves may also leak blood back into the atrium, producing a sound called a murmur. Mitral valve prolapse is a benign condition that rarely requires treatment.

Left atrium
Prolapsed valve
Normal valve (closed)
Left ventricle

The Aging Heart

Aortic Valve

Cross-Section of Electrical Conduction Tissue

Fibrous tissue accumulation

Sclerosis

Endocardium of left atrium thickened and opaque
Endocardium of ventricles is thinner

Cross-Section of Ventricular Heart Muscle

Fibrosis
Lipofuscin accumulation
Basophilic material accumulation
Fat accumulation

©2008 Wolters Kluwer Health | Lippincott Williams & Wilkins | Published by Anatomical Chart Company, Skokie, IL

Understanding Hypertension

What Is Hypertension?

Hypertension is the result of persistent high arterial blood pressure which may cause damage to the vessels and arteries of the heart, brain, kidneys and eyes. The entire circulatory system is affected since it becomes increasingly more difficult for the blood to travel from the heart to the major organs. Multiple blood pressure readings are taken to establish an average and analyzed by a physician to determine hypertension.

What Causes Hypertension?

Modern life styles tend to increase blood pressure causing hypertension. Some of the known factors include a high salt intake, excessive alcohol consumption and obesity. Genetic factors may also influence this disease. Primary hypertension is the most common type and it generally is improved by a healthier life style; and medication when needed. Secondary hypertension is the result of a disorder or abnormality of the kidney, adrenal gland or other vital organ. This less common type of hypertension is often treated surgically. Hypertension may also occur during pregnancy and requires special attention.

What Is Blood Pressure?

Blood pressure is a measure of the pressure of the blood against the walls of the arteries. It is dependent upon the action of the heart, the elasticity of the artery walls and the volume and thickness of the blood. The blood pressure readings are a ratio of the maximum or systolic pressure (as the heart pushes the blood out to the body) written over the minimum or diastolic pressure (as the heart begins to fill with blood).

$$\frac{\text{Systolic pressure}}{\text{Diastolic pressure}} \quad \text{or} \quad \frac{120}{80}$$

Symptoms of Hypertension

You may have:
NO SYMPTOMS!
(No noticeable symptoms may be felt even with high blood pressure)

or you may have:
Headaches
Blurring of vision
Chest pain
Frequent urination at night

Effects in Blood Vessels

Increase in arterial blood pressure can change and damage the inside artery wall. The wall may become thicker while the space which transports the blood becomes smaller (vascular hypertrophy).

Adventitia
External elastic membrane
Media
Internal elastic Membrane
Lamina propria
Endothelium
Lumen

Normal Blood Vessel

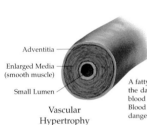

Adventitia
Enlarged Media (smooth muscle)
Small Lumen

Vascular Hypertrophy

A fatty build up, also called plaque, develops in the damaged arterial wall, clogging the flow of blood throughout the artery (atherosclerosis). Blood clots may form more easily and become dangerous if dislodged.

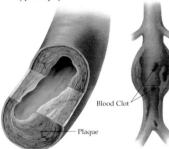

Blood Clot
Plaque

Atherosclerosis

Under increasing blood pressure, a weakening of the artery wall may balloon out (aneurysm) and break, causing blood loss, tissue damage and even death.

Effects in the Brain

Hypertension is the major cause of stroke. The harmful effects of hypertension in the brain may be caused by blood clots stopping blood flow to parts of the brain. Aneurysms may burst under increasing pressure causing hemorrhage and damage to brain tissue.

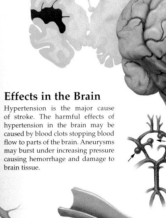

Blood clot

Aneurysm

Effects in the Eye

A thorough eye examination by a physician may lead to the diagnosis of hypertension. This can be determined by the vascular changes in the back of the eye (retina).

Effects in the Kidneys

The kidneys are easily damaged by hypertension. In addition, many kidney diseases cause hypertension. Increased blood pressure disrupts the kidneys' ability to regulate salt and water balance in the body which can make hypertension worse.

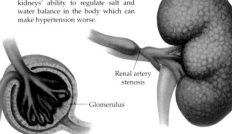

Renal artery stenosis
Glomerulus

Blood Flow in the Heart

The right side of the heart receives blood from the body and delivers this unoxygenated blood to the lungs. The left side of the heart receives oxygen rich blood from the lungs and pumps it through the arteries to all organs and tissues in the body.

Normal Heart

Right ventricle   Left ventricle

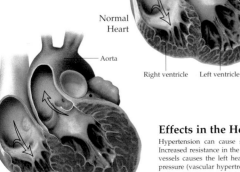

Aorta

Left Ventricular Hypertrophy

Effects in the Heart

Hypertension can cause serious health problems to this vital organ. Increased resistance in the arteries, due to stiffness and narrowing of the vessels causes the left heart to work harder pumping against a higher pressure (vascular hypertrophy). The left ventricle may become enlarged and unable to respond to this pressure increase. In addition, the heart muscle may suffer from decreased blood flow due to atherosclerosis of the small arteries of the heart.

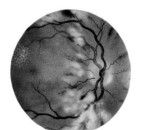

Healthy Life Style Changes

Decrease your blood pressure by:
• Reducing body weight
• Restricting dietary salt
• Increasing fiber and decreasing fat in your diet
• Not smoking
• Avoiding excess alcohol
• Exercising regularly
• Developing relaxation techniques

It is very important to follow your physician's instructions and to take any medications as prescribed.

©2008 Wolters Kluwer Health | Lippincott Williams & Wilkins | Published by Anatomical Chart Company, Skokie, IL

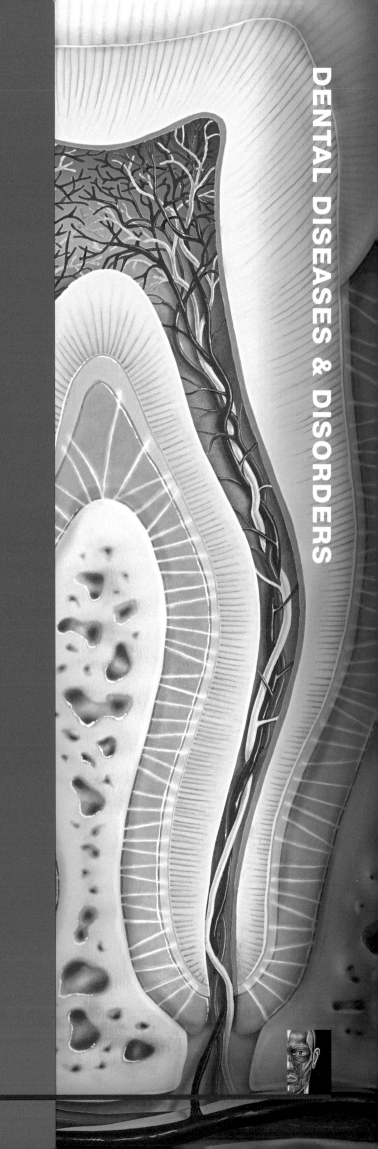

• Disorders of the Teeth and Jaw • Temporomandibular Joint (TMJ)

Disorders of the Teeth and Jaw

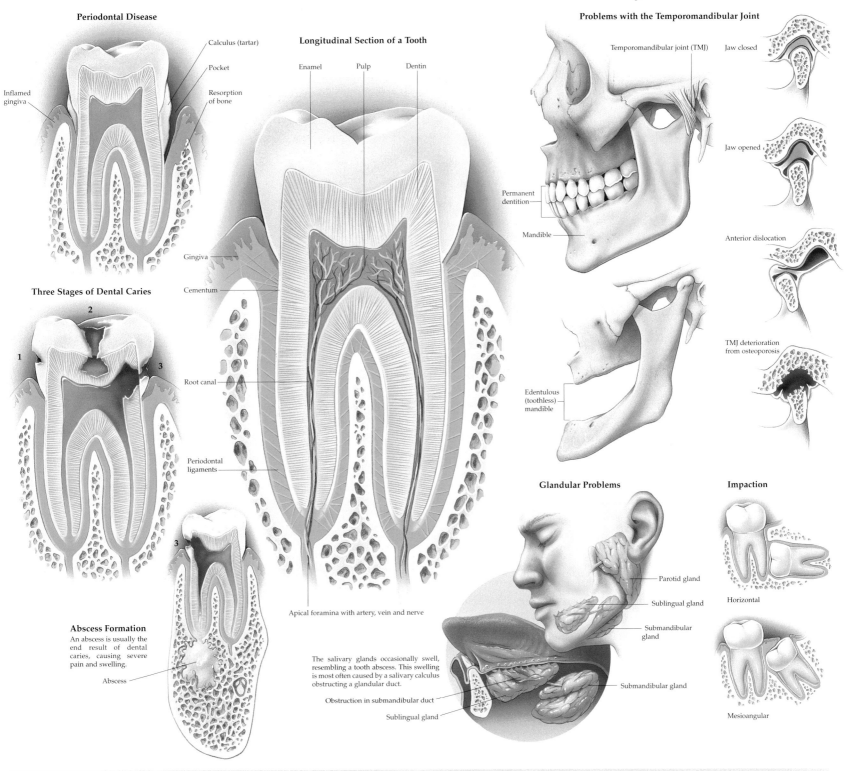

Periodontal Disease

- Calculus (tartar)
- Pocket
- Resorption of bone
- Inflamed gingiva

Longitudinal Section of a Tooth

- Enamel
- Pulp
- Dentin
- Gingiva
- Cementum
- Root canal
- Periodontal ligaments
- Apical foramina with artery, vein and nerve

Three Stages of Dental Caries

1
2
3

3

Abscess Formation

An abscess is usually the end result of dental caries, causing severe pain and swelling.

- Abscess

Problems with the Temporomandibular Joint

- Temporomandibular joint (TMJ)
- Jaw closed
- Jaw opened
- Anterior dislocation
- TMJ deterioration from osteoporosis
- Permanent dentition
- Mandible
- Edentulous (toothless) mandible

Glandular Problems

The salivary glands occasionally swell, resembling a tooth abscess. This swelling is most often caused by a salivary calculus obstructing a glandular duct.

- Parotid gland
- Sublingual gland
- Submandibular gland
- Submandibular gland
- Obstruction in submandibular duct
- Sublingual gland

Impaction

- Horizontal
- Mesioangular

Dental Anomalies

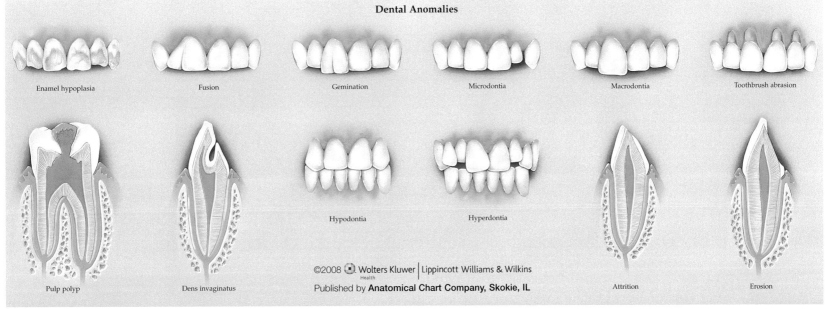

- Enamel hypoplasia
- Fusion
- Gemination
- Microdontia
- Macrodontia
- Toothbrush abrasion
- Pulp polyp
- Dens invaginatus
- Hypodontia
- Hyperdontia
- Attrition
- Erosion

©2008 Wolters Kluwer | Lippincott Williams & Wilkins
Health
Published by **Anatomical Chart Company**, Skokie, IL

Key: Muscles (m.)

A. Temporalis m.
B. Temporomandibular joint
C. Masseter m.
D. Stylohyoid m.
E. Digastric m. (posterior belly)
F. Longus capitis m.
G. Levator scapulae m.
H. Trapezius m.
I. Posterior scalene m.
J. Middle scalene m.
K. Sternocleidomastoid m.
L. Inferior pharyngeal constrictor m.
M. Thyrohyoid m.
N. Sternothyroid m.
O. Omohyoid m.
P. Sternohyoid m.
Q. Hyoglossus m.
R. Mylohyoid m.
S. Digastric m. (anterior belly)

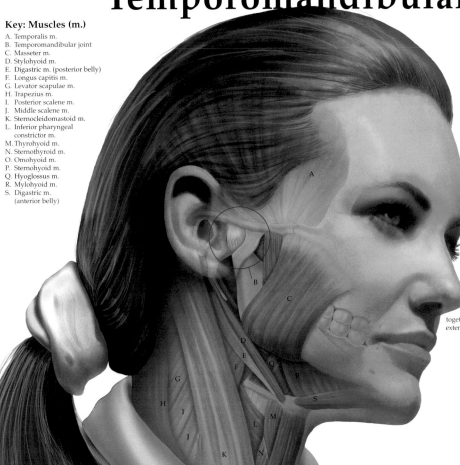

Normal Jaw (closed)

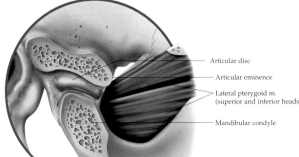

Articular disc
Articular eminence
Lateral pterygoid m. (superior and inferior heads)
Mandibular condyle

What is TMJ Syndrome?

TMJ syndrome is a term often used to describe a disorder of the temporomandibular joints (jaw joints) and/or the muscles that control the joints and balance the head on the spinal column. It is a collection of symptoms that occur when the jaw joints and/or surrounding muscles do not work together properly. The problem also can extend down the neck and back.

Normal Jaw (open)

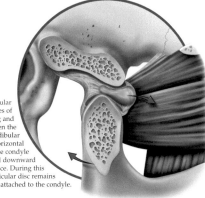

The purpose of the articular disc is to cushion the bones of the TMJ during opening and closing of the mouth. When the mouth opens, the mandibular condyle rotates on a horizontal axis. At the same time, the condyle and disc glide forward and downward on the articular eminence. During this entire motion the articular disc remains attached to the condyle.

Nerves of the Temporomandibular Region

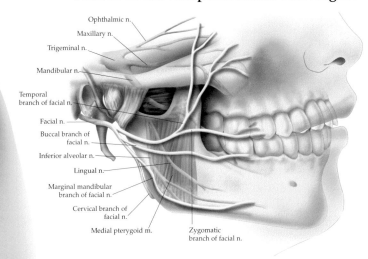

Ophthalmic n.
Maxillary n.
Trigeminal n.
Mandibular n.
Temporal branch of facial n.
Facial n.
Buccal branch of facial n.
Inferior alveolar n.
Lingual n.
Marginal mandibular branch of facial n.
Cervical branch of facial n.
Medial pterygoid m.
Zygomatic branch of facial n.

Common TMJ Syndrome Causes and Disorders

Whiplash

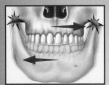

Whiplash causes the muscles of the neck to be jarred and pulled violently, often resulting in ligament tears, stretching of structures to their limits and discal tearing. All can lead to the development of TMJ symptoms.

Malocclusion

Malocclusion is the abnormal contact of opposing teeth with respect to the temporomandibular joint that interferes with the efficient movement of the jaw during mastication. It is one of the most frequent triggers of TMJ syndrome. Malocclusion, even on a minute scale can trigger the spasm of muscles, resulting in pain.

Bruxism/Clenching

Bruxism, the grinding of teeth, usually occurs during sleep. Clenching can occur throughout the day or night. Both can be directly related to TMJ, either as a trigger for muscle spasms or as a result of malocclusion. Constant grinding also causes pressure on the TMJ. Bruxing can put pressure on the articular disc, squeezing out synovial fluid and robbing it of lubrication.

Systemic Diseases

The TMJ, like any other joint, is susceptible to any of the systemic diseases. Immune disorders such as osteoarthritis, rheumatoid arthritis, psoriatic arthritis and systemic lupus erythematosus and electrolyte imbalances can produce inflammation and muscle cramping in the TMJ. In addition, viral infections can cause damage to the surfaces of the TMJ.

Loss of Teeth

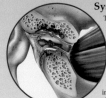

When a tooth is lost, the teeth around it tend to shift to fill the space. This change can alter the way the teeth gear in relation to the joint, causing symptoms to develop.

Disc Displacement

The jaw joint, in addition to being a ball and socket joint, glides forward and backward. When functioning correctly, the articular cartilage lies between the condyle head of the mandible and the roof of the joint. It normally follows the condylar head in its forward and backward movement. If the ligaments that hold the disc to the condylar head are injured, the disc can slip out of place and can no longer serve as a normal cushion between the lower and upper parts of the jaw. Typically, the disc is pulled forward. Mild displacements can cause a clicking or popping sound in the joint and sometimes can be painful. Permanent damage may result from the displacements.

Symptoms

Extracapsular- Outside the jaw joint.

- Headaches
- Tooth pain (caused by bruxism)
- Numbness or tingling of fingers
- Dizziness

- Neck, shoulder or back pain
- Pain behind eyes
- Earaches or ringing in ears

Intracapsular- Within the jaw joint.

- Crepitus (grinding sound)
- Clicking or popping

- Locking or limited range of motion
- Pain in and around jaw joints

Disorders Sometimes Mistaken for TMJ Syndrome

- Migraine headache
- Chemical allergies
- Temporal tendinitis
- Psychosomatic headache

- Ernest syndrome
- Sinusitis
- Brain tumors
- Trauma

Treatment

Phase 1- Attempts to break the cycle of muscle spasms, thereby relieving pain and producing a physiological relationship between the maxilla and mandible. Treatments can include:

- Use of an intra-oral orthotic or splint
- Anti-inflammatory medications
- Stress management

- Physical therapy
- Muscle relaxants
- Manipulative treatment

Phase 2- Attempts to break the cycle of pain through more permanent means of treatment. Treatments can include:

- Adjustment of dental occlusion
- Orthodontics
- Reconstruction of teeth

- Orthognathic surgery (surgical relocation of teeth or jaw)
- Replacement of missing teeth
- Surgery on TMJ itself (last resort)

©2008 Wolters Kluwer Health | Lippincott Williams & Wilkins I Published by **Anatomical Chart Company, Skokie, IL**

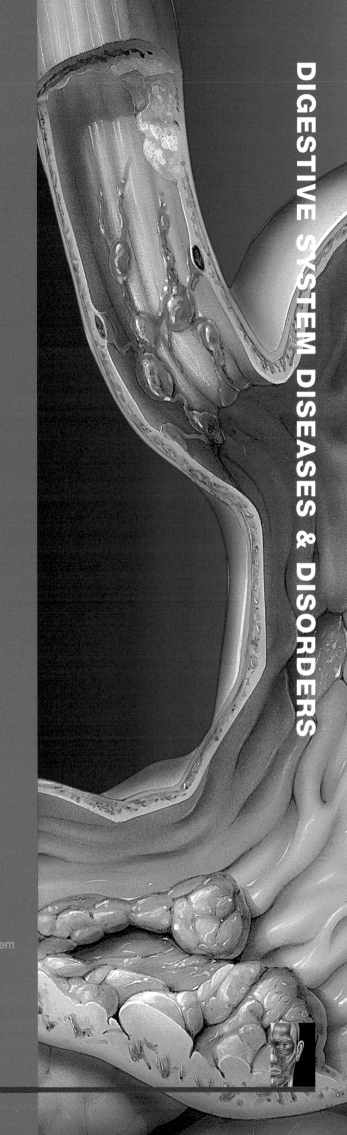

Gastroesophageal Disorders and Digestive Anatomy

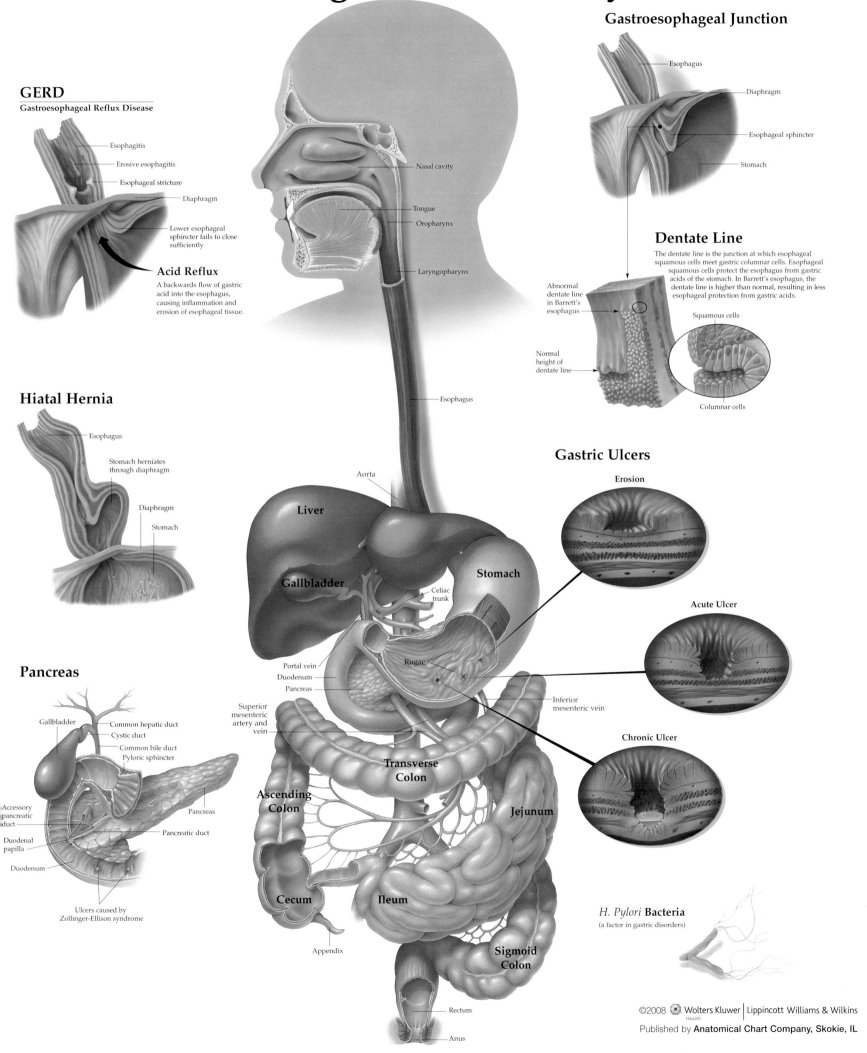

Gastroesophageal Junction

Esophagus

Diaphragm

Esophageal sphincter

Stomach

GERD
Gastroesophageal Reflux Disease

Esophagitis

Erosive esophagitis

Esophageal stricture

Diaphragm

Lower esophageal sphincter fails to close sufficiently

Acid Reflux

A backwards flow of gastric acid into the esophagus, causing inflammation and erosion of esophageal tissue.

Dentate Line

The dentate line is the junction at which esophageal squamous cells meet gastric columnar cells. Esophageal squamous cells protect the esophagus from gastric acids of the stomach. In Barrett's esophagus, the dentate line is higher than normal, resulting in less esophageal protection from gastric acids.

Abnormal dentate line in Barrett's esophagus

Normal height of dentate line

Squamous cells

Columnar cells

Nasal cavity

Tongue

Oropharynx

Laryngopharynx

Esophagus

Hiatal Hernia

Esophagus

Stomach herniates through diaphragm

Diaphragm

Stomach

Gastric Ulcers

Erosion

Acute Ulcer

Chronic Ulcer

Aorta

Liver

Gallbladder

Celiac trunk

Stomach

Portal vein

Duodenum

Pancreas

Rugae

Inferior mesenteric vein

Superior mesenteric artery and vein

Pancreas

Gallbladder

Common hepatic duct

Cystic duct

Common bile duct

Pyloric sphincter

Accessory pancreatic duct

Pancreas

Duodenal papilla

Pancreatic duct

Duodenum

Ulcers caused by Zollinger-Ellison syndrome

Transverse Colon

Ascending Colon

Jejunum

Cecum

Ileum

Appendix

Sigmoid Colon

H. Pylori **Bacteria**
(a factor in gastric disorders)

Rectum

Anus

©2008 Wolters Kluwer | Lippincott Williams & Wilkins
Health

Published by Anatomical Chart Company, Skokie, IL

Diseases of the Digestive System

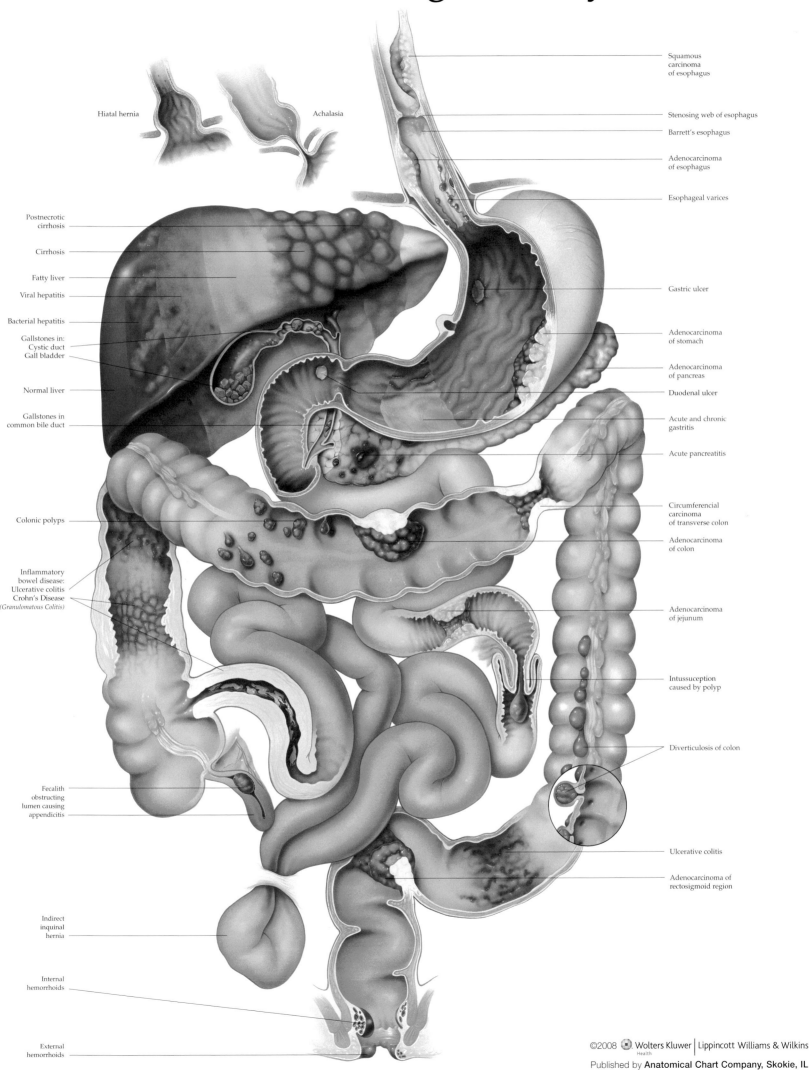

Hiatal hernia

Achalasia

Squamous carcinoma of esophagus

Stenosing web of esophagus

Barrett's esophagus

Adenocarcinoma of esophagus

Esophageal varices

Postnecrotic cirrhosis

Cirrhosis

Fatty liver

Viral hepatitis

Bacterial hepatitis

Gallstones in:
Cystic duct
Gall bladder

Normal liver

Gallstones in common bile duct

Gastric ulcer

Adenocarcinoma of stomach

Adenocarcinoma of pancreas

Duodenal ulcer

Acute and chronic gastritis

Acute pancreatitis

Colonic polyps

Inflammatory bowel disease:
Ulcerative colitis
Crohn's Disease
(Granulomatous Colitis)

Circumferencial carcinoma of transverse colon

Adenocarcinoma of colon

Adenocarcinoma of jejunum

Intussuception caused by polyp

Diverticulosis of colon

Fecalith obstructing lumen causing appendicitis

Ulcerative colitis

Adenocarcinoma of rectosigmoid region

Indirect inquinal hernia

Internal hemorrhoids

External hemorrhoids

©2008 Wolters Kluwer | Lippincott Williams & Wilkins
Health

Published by **Anatomical Chart Company, Skokie, IL**

Understanding Ulcers

What is an Ulcer?

An ulcer is a lesion on the mucous surface of the esophagus, stomach or duodenum caused by inflammation that progressively erodes the superficial tissues. Millions of people are affected with ulcers every year.

Esophagus
Stomach
Duodenum

Esophagus

Longitudinal muscle
Circular muscle
Submucosa
Muscularis mucosa
Blood vessels
Mucosa

Duodenum

Serosa
Longitudinal muscle
Circular muscle
Submucosa
Blood vessels
Villus
Muscularis mucosa
Mucosa
Kerckring's valve

Pylorus
Incisura
Antrum

Stomach

Serosa
Blood vessel
Gastric pits
Longitudinal muscle
Circular muscle
Oblique muscle
Submucosa
Muscularis mucosa
Mucosa

Esophageal ulcer
"Z-Z" line
Fundus
Body
Rugae

What Causes Ulcers?

pH 2 (acid)
pH 7 (base)
pH gradient

Gastric Pit
Acid Flow

Bicarbonate flux
Fenestrated capillary

Chief cells (produce mucus)

Bicarbonate flux

Parietal cells (produce stomach acid, HCl, Bicarbonate)

Ulcers can be caused by irritants such as alcohol and drugs, an imbalance of gastric acids, and bacteria that inflame mucosal tissues.

Types of Ulcers

Erosion

Penetration of only the superficial layer

Mucosa
Muscularis mucosa
Submucosa
Oblique muscle
Circular muscle
Longitudinal muscle
Serosa

Acute Ulcer

Penetration into the muscular layer

Ulcers may occur anywhere in the stomach, duodenum or esophagus. The crater of an ulcer may penetrate different layers of tissues. If this damage is recurring or if healing does not take place, the crater may penetrate the entire wall and into adjacent tissues and organs, like the pancreas. As with most ulcers, scarring causes puckering so that mucosal folds are seen to radiate outward in a spoke-like formation.

Perforating Ulcer

Penetration of wall creating a passage for gastric acids, other fluids and air to enter adjacent spaces of the body.

Exudate
Granulation tissue

A Closer Look

Helicobacter pylori

Chemical Irritant

Helicobacter pylori

Lamellipodia

Growing blood vessels
Gastric pit
Basal lamina
Mucous neck cells

Bacteria have been found to be a contributing factor in chronic gastritis (chronic inflammation of stomach mucosa) and in ulcer formation. Tiny *Helicobacter pylori* are typically seen within the muscular layers and between cells that line the gastric pits. The bacteria cause inflammation of these tissues which can lead to ulcers. Treatment with acid-reducing medication and antibiotics can reduce the recurrence of this process.

In the absence of an effective mucous barrier, an irritant such as excess stomach acid can cause the basal lamina to be sloughed off. This process is called *exfoliation*. Normally, a process called *rapid reepithelialization* replenishes the damaged epithelium and repairs any defects.

How Ulcers Heal

Mucus-secreting surface cells

Exfoliation

As exfoliation occurs within the stomach mucosa, the epithelial cells that line the stomach and cover the basal lamina become damaged. This exposes the underlying basal lamina to the irritants, causing it to detach and be sloughed off.

Restitution

Rapid reepithelialization occurs constantly and normally, repairing stomach tissues. The mucous neck cells that line the gastric pits divide at a rapid rate and send out lamellipodia, or thin feet, that move up to cover the regenerating basal lamina.

Recovery

The mucous neck cells transform back into more typical cuboidal surface cells, and the normal architecture of the basal lamina is restored.

©2008 Wolters Kluwer Health | Lippincott Williams & Wilkins

Published by Anatomical Chart Company, Skokie, IL

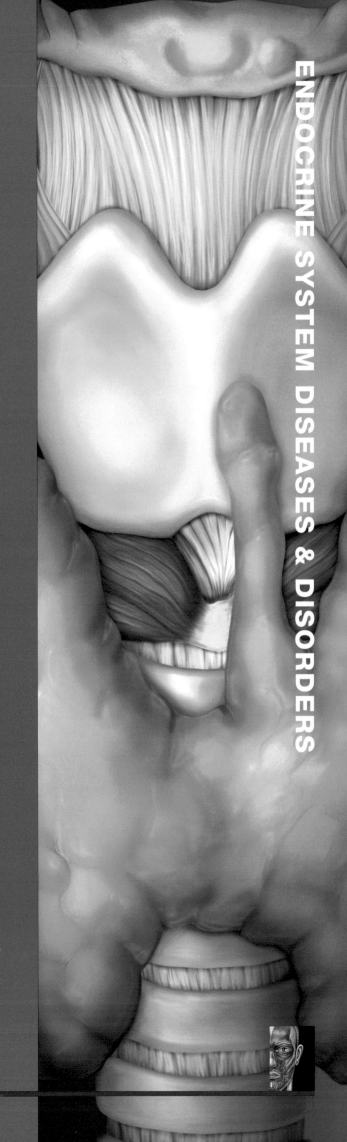

ENDOCRINE SYSTEM DISEASES & DISORDERS

• Understanding Type 1 Diabetes • Understanding Type 2 Diabetes • Metabolic Syndrome
• Thyroid Disorders

Understanding Type 1 Diabetes

Pancreas

Insulin molecules (from pancreas)

As food enters the digestive system, it is broken down into glucose. It is either stored in the liver or absorbed into the bloodstream, where it is used by the body for energy.

Normally, in response to a rise in blood glucose levels, the pancreas releases insulin. In Type 1 diabetes, the pancreas produces little or no insulin.

Glucose molecules (from digestive system)

Normal Body Cell

Normally, insulin molecules bind to the body's cell receptors. When activated by insulin, portals open to allow glucose to enter the cells and be converted to energy.

Body Cell with Diabetes

Without insulin, portals do not open. As a result, glucose builds up in the blood and is not able to enter the cells to be converted to energy.

Blood vessel

Red blood cells

Opened glucose portal

Insulin receptor

Closed glucose portal

Glucose converted to energy

Energy-deprived cell

Glucose molecule

Red blood cell

What is Type 1 Diabetes?

Type 1 diabetes occurs when the pancreas produces little or no insulin which is needed to process glucose. The body's immune system attacks or destroys the beta cells that secrete insulin.

- Glucose, also known as blood sugar, is the body's main source of fuel.
- Insulin is needed to transport glucose from the bloodstream into the other cells of the body for energy

A person with Type 1 diabetes is producing little to no insulin; as a result, the glucose (blood sugar) builds up in the bloodstream and can cause complications in the rest of the body.

Most people develop Type 1 diabetes when they are children or young adults, but it can occur at any age.

Controlling Type 1 Diabetes

Diabetes control means keeping the level of glucose in the blood as close to normal as possible. People with diabetes need to maintain a balance between medication, diet, and exercise.

There is no cure or prevention for Type 1 Diabetes as yet. Controlling this disease requires the assistance of a medical diabetes team; it also includes:

- Taking insulin.
- Adhering to a prescribed meal plan with carbohydrate counting.
- Brushing and flossing teeth and gums regularly.
- Visiting the doctor regularly, including an ophthalmologist and dentist.
- Self-monitoring of blood glucose.
- Exercising regularly.
- Checking for sores, cuts, and blisters on feet.
- Not smoking.

Risk Factors
It is unclear what causes Type 1 diabetes; a combination of genetic and environmental factors is thought to be responsible.

Short-term Complications

Hypoglycemia
(low-blood sugar) can develop quickly in people with diabetes.

Symptoms include:
- Weakness/dizziness
- Sweating
- Nervousness
- Loss of coordination
- Hunger
- Inability to concentrate
- Shaking
- Headache
- Pale skin color
- Seizure
- Loss of consciousness

Hyperglycemia
(high blood sugar) can develop slowly, at times, over a period of days.

Symptoms include:
- Frequent urination
- High levels of sugar in the urine
- Increased thirst

Ketoacidosis
is another dangerous complication of Type 1 diabetes. It occurs when there is not enough insulin in the body and ketones (fat bodies) build up to a poisonous level in the blood, which consequently shows up in the urine. This condition can build up slowly and can lead to a diabetic coma or even death. The first symptoms of ketoacidosis are similar to those of hyperglycemia, but additional symptoms include:

- Constant fatigue
- Dry skin and mouth
- Stomach pain
- Fruity or sweet-smelling breath
- Flushed face
- Nausea and vomiting
- Deep/rapid breathing (shortness of breath)
- Inability to pay attention/confusion

Long-term Complications

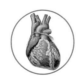

Eye Complications
High blood glucose levels can affect blood vessels in the eyes; over time, this can lead to vision loss or blindness.
- Diabetic Retinopathy occurs when one of the arteries that supplies blood to the retina becomes blocked. Blood flow diminishes, which can lead to blindness.
- Glaucoma occurs when the buildup of fluid in the eye causes increased pressure, which can damage sight perception.
- Cataracts are the clouding of the normally transparent lenses of the eye, which can result in fuzzy vision.

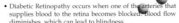

Heart Disease
People with diabetes are at high risk for diseases of the heart and blood vessels, such as heart attack and stroke. It is especially important for people with diabetes to keep blood pressure and cholesterol at healthy levels.

Kidney Disease (Nephropathy)
High levels of blood glucose can damage the glomeruli (the filtering units of the kidney), which can reduce the kidney's ability to remove waste and retain important nutrients such as protein.

Gum Disease and Oral Complications
Diabetes increases the risk of gum disease and mouth infections. The rise in the blood glucose level can make mouth infections worse.

Nerve Damage (Neuropathy)
High levels of blood glucose can damage the nerves. These nerves run throughout the body, connecting the brain and spinal cord to the rest of the body. Symptoms of possible nerve damage are tingling, pain, numbness, or weakness in feet or hands with an unawareness of feelings. Neuropathy decreases the ability of a person with diabetes to feel the warning pain of infection.

Foot Complications
In combination with neuropathy, poor blood circulation can lead to ulcers and infections on the feet that do not heal. These problems can eventually result in gangrene and amputation.

Understanding Type 2 Diabetes

36

Pancreas

Glucose molecules (from digestive system)

Insulin molecules (from pancreas)

Normally, in response to a rise in blood glucose levels, the pancreas releases insulin. In Type 2 diabetes, problems occur when the insulin that is produced doesn't work or when the body's cells resist insulin.

Blood vessel

Normal Body Cell
Normally, insulin molecules bind to the body's cell receptors. When activated by insulin, portals open to allow glucose to enter the cells, where it is converted to energy.

Body Cell with Diabetes
In Type 2 diabetes, the body's cells develop a resistance to insulin, making it more difficult for glucose to enter the cell.

Opened glucose portal

Insulin receptor

Closed glucose portal

Glucose converted to energy

Energy-deprived cell

Red blood cells

As a result of Type 2 diabetes, cells don't get enough energy. This causes glucose to build up in the blood vessels, resulting in damage to all body organs.

Symptoms

Symptoms of Type 2 diabetes usually develop gradually and may not appear until many years after the onset of the disease. They include:

- Frequent urination
- Excessive thirst
- Fatigue
- Very dry skin
- Sores that are slow to heal
- More infections than usual
- Tingling or numbness in the hands
- Dehydration
- Unexplained weight loss
- Extreme hunger
- Sudden vision change

Some people with diabetes do not have any symptoms.

Risk Factors

- Older age
- Overweight or obesity
- Pre-diabetes: blood glucose levels that are higher than normal but not yet high enough to be diagnosed as diabetes
- Family history of diabetes
- Prior history of gestational diabetes
- Physical inactivity/lack of exercise
- Race/ethnicity (African Americans, Hispanic Americans, Native Americans, and Asian Americans are almost twice as likely as Caucasian Americans to develop Type 2 diabetes).

Controlling Diabetes

People with diabetes can prevent or delay problems by keeping blood glucose, blood pressure, and cholesterol under control and getting regular medical care.

Diabetes control means keeping the level of sugar (glucose) in the blood as close to normal as possible. People with diabetes need to work with a health care team to maintain a balance between medication, blood sugar monitoring, diet, and exercise.

These seven things should be done every day to help control your diabetes:
- Follow the healthy meal plan recommended by your health care provider or nutritionist.
- Become more physically active.
- Brush your teeth and gums and floss.
- Don't smoke.
- Check your feet for cuts, blisters, or sores.
- Take your diabetes medicine.
- Check your blood glucose.

What Is Type 2 Diabetes?

With Type 2 diabetes, the body either can't make enough insulin or the insulin doesn't work as it should.

- Glucose, also known as a sugar, is the body's main source of fuel.
- Insulin is needed to help glucose get from the bloodstream to the other cells of the body.

In Type 2 diabetes, the glucose can't get into the cells because the insulin is not working correctly. This causes the sugar (glucose) to stay in the bloodstream, leading to a high blood sugar level. Too much sugar in the blood can cause serious health problems unless it is treated.

Complications

Without proper management, long-term diabetes can damage many parts of the body, such as the eyes, mouth, cardiovascular system, kidneys, hand and feet, and nerves.

Heart Disease and Stroke
Poor blood glucose control, high blood pressure, and high blood fats (cholesterol) can damage arteries leading to heart attack or stroke.

Vascular Disease
Poor diabetes control can cause circulation problems in the blood vessels of the legs and feet. This also can affect the healing of wounds and infections. In extreme situations, gangrene can develop and amputations can be necessary.

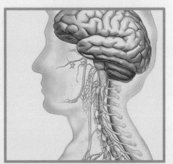

Nerve Damage (Neuropathy)
In diabetic neuropathy (nerve damage), nerves that branch from the brain and spinal cord to the rest of the body are damaged as a result of high blood glucose. Symptoms of possible nerve damage are burning sensations in the toes that eventually progresses up the foot.

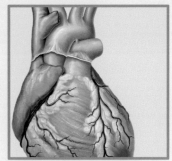

Kidney Disease (Nephropathy)
High blood glucose affects small blood vessels in the glomeruli (the filtering units of the kidney). Damage to these vessels (glomeruli) reduces the kidney's ability to remove waste and to reserve important nutrients such as protein.

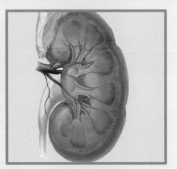

Periodontal Disease
Diabetes increases the risk of gum disease and mouth infections. This can make blood glucose levels rise, which in turn can make mouth infections worse.

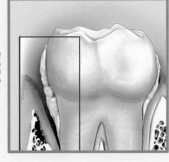

Eye Disease
High blood glucose levels can affect blood vessels in the eyes. Over time, this can lead to vision loss or blindness.

Glaucoma
Glaucoma, the buildup of fluid in the eye, causes increased pressure and can damage sight perception.

Cataracts
A cataract is the clouding of the normally transparent lens of the eye, which results in fuzzy vision.

Diabetic Retinopathy
When one of the arteries that supplies blood to the retina becomes blocked, blood flow diminishes which can lead to blindness.

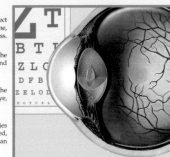

37

Metabolic Syndrome

What is Metabolic Syndrome?

Metabolic syndrome describes a common condition in which **obesity, high blood pressure, high blood glucose ("blood sugar"),** and an **abnormal cholesterol profile (dyslipidemia)** cluster together in one person. When these risk factors occur together, the chance of developing **coronary heart disease, stroke,** and **diabetes** is much greater than when these risk factors develop independently. According to the American Heart Association, almost 25% of Americans are affected by metabolic syndrome.

Metabolic Syndrome Risk Factors

To be diagnosed with metabolic syndrome, patients need to have at least **three** of the following risk factors:

Obesity

Obesity is defined as having too much body fat. A person is considered obese when his/her weight is 20% or more above ideal weight. Obesity promotes insulin resistance, an inability to respond normally to insulin. People with fat situated mainly around the stomach (abdomen) are considered **"apple-shaped."** They have a higher risk of many of the serious conditions associated with metabolic syndrome. Ask your healthcare provider what your ideal weight should be.

Apple-shaped:
Excess fat mostly around the abdomen.

<u>Metabolic Syndrome Risk Factor:</u>
Waist measurement greater than
35 inches (women) or 40 inches (men)

High Blood Glucose

Sugar (glucose) is what supplies the body with energy. Normally, this sugar (glucose) is rapidly cleared from the blood and stored as energy. If sugar stays in the blood it causes an unhealthy buildup called **high blood glucose**. Glucose in the blood reaches all of the body's organs and systems, including the heart, arteries and veins, kidneys, and nervous system. This constant "sugar-attack" has the same affect as eating too much candy and not brushing your teeth--it causes organ system decay or degeneration. People with high blood glucose are at risk for many diseases including heart attack, stroke, blindness, and amputation. High blood glucose levels (or pre-diabetes) often leads to the development of type 2 diabetes.

<u>Metabolic Syndrome Risk Factor:</u>
Glucose of at least 110 mg/dL or greater

High Blood Pressure

Blood pressure is the force that helps the blood flow through the blood vessels. When the blood pressure in the arteries is too high, it is called **high blood pressure.** High blood pressure damages blood vessels. If blood vessels are subjected to high blood pressure for an extended period of time, they thicken, and become less flexible. This is called **arteriosclerosis**, and it can affect the arteries that supply blood to the heart.

Blood pressure is measured using two numbers. The first number, called **systolic pressure**, is measured just after the heart contracts and the pressure is greatest. The second number is **diastolic pressure**. It is measured when the heart relaxes and the pressure is lowest.

Normal blood pressure is about 110/75 mmHg. High blood pressure alone causes no symptoms, but it does increase the risk of heart attack, stroke, and kidney failure.

<u>Metabolic Syndrome Risk Factor:</u>
Blood pressure greater than 130/85 mmHg

Abnormal Cholesterol Profile (Dyslipidemia)

Cholesterol is a type of fat in your blood. Cholesterol either comes from the foods you eat or is made by your liver. It is found in all of the body's cells. There are "good" and "bad" types of cholesterol. Too much of the "bad" cholesterol (triglycerides and LDL) and not enough "good" cholesterol (HDL) can increase your risk of coronary heart disease. Triglycerides and HDL levels are important indicators of metabolic syndrome.

Triglycerides

High triglyceride levels in the blood can help clog the arteries with fatty deposits called plaque (atherosclerosis), making it difficult for oxygen-rich blood to reach the heart. High triglyceride levels increase your risk of having a heart attack.

<u>Metabolic Syndrome Risk Factor:</u>
Triglyceride level greater than 150 mg/dL

HDL Cholesterol

HDL cholesterol (the "good cholesterol") helps remove deposits from within the blood vessels and it stops the blood vessels from becoming blocked. The more HDL in your blood, the better it is for your heart. When HDL cholesterol levels are low, there is a greater risk of developing a heart attack or stroke.

<u>Metabolic Syndrome Risk Factor:</u>
HDL cholesterol level less than 50 mg/dL (women)
and less than 40 mg/dL (men

Organs Affected by Untreated Metabolic Syndrome

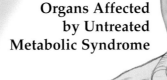

A Brain

High blood glucose:
Sugar (glucose) builds up in bloodstream.

B Heart

C Pancreas

High blood pressure,
if not treated causes damage to the lining of the arteries.

Fibrous plaque (atherosclerosis)

Medical Conditions Associated with Metabolic Syndrome

People with untreated metabolic syndrome are at a higher risk of cardiovascular disease (such as coronary heart disease and stroke) and type 2 diabetes.

A **Stroke**

The term stroke refers to the sudden death of brain tissue caused by a lack of oxygen to the brain. In ischemic stroke, blood flow to an area of the brain is either blocked or reduced. This blockage may result from atherosclerosis and blood clot formation.

B **Coronary Heart Disease**

Narrowing of the arteries in the heart usually causes coronary heart disease which can lead to heart attacks. The buildup of plaque in the lining of the arteries (atherosclerosis) can cause this narrowing. All of the metabolic syndrome risk factors can result in atherosclerosis. Heart attacks occur when blood cannot flow through the clogged arteries. As a result, the heart does not get enough oxygen and stops working.

C **Type 2 Diabetes**

Type 2 diabetes is a disease in which the pancreas produces little or no insulin and/or the body loses the ability to respond normally to insulin (insulin resistance). Insulin is needed to transport glucose into the cells for use as energy. Without insulin, body tissues have less access to essential nutrients for energy and storage. Without proper management, diabetes can lead to complications that affect the eyes, mouth, cardiovascular system, kidneys, nerves, and extremities.

What Causes Metabolic Syndrome?

Some studies suggest that metabolic syndrome is closely tied to an individual's metabolism, or how the body processes food. Normally, food is absorbed into the bloodstream in the form of sugar (glucose) and other basic substances. When glucose levels in the bloodstream rise, the pancreas (an organ behind the stomach) releases a hormone called insulin. Insulin attaches to the body's cells allowing glucose to enter, where it is used for energy. In some people, the body's cells are not able to respond to insulin (insulin resistance).

It is this condition of insulin resistance that some studies suggest is behind the development of metabolic syndrome.

How is Metabolic Syndrome Treated?

Metabolic syndrome is a disease that requires long-term management of each of the risk factors. Poor nutrition, and lack of exercise are underlying causes of these risk factors. It has been shown that with lifestyle changes and treatment, including medications, people with metabolic syndrome can greatly decrease their chances of developing serious complications. Regular monitoring of blood pressure, cholesterol, and glucose are important to detect the syndrome. Even though you may feel fine, you may still have risk factors of metabolic syndrome. It is important to know your numbers and discuss them with your doctor.

Treatment options usually include the following:

• **Weight loss-**
If you are obese, a weight loss of 5 to 10% of your body weight can help your body regain its ability to recognize insulin.

• **Exercise-**
Increased activity reverses insulin resistance. It also helps lower blood pressure, lower "bad" cholesterol, raise "good" cholesterol levels and reduce the risk of developing type 2 diabetes.

• **Eat a heart healthy diet-**
Reduce saturated fat, cholesterol, and salt intake. Increase intake of high fiber foods like fruits, vegetables, and grains.

©2008 Wolters Kluwer Health | Lippincott Williams & Wilkins | Published by Anatomical Chart Company, Skokie, IL

38

Thyroid Disorders

What Is the Thyroid?

The thyroid is a small gland that is wrapped around the windpipe (trachea), just below the thyroid cartilage. The thyroid plays an important role in health and affects every organ, tissue, and cell in the body. It makes hormones that maintain the normal function of many organ systems and regulate metabolism (how the body uses and stores energy from foods eaten).

When the thyroid is not working properly (called thyroid disorder), it can affect:

- Body weight
- Energy level
- Sleeping patterns
- Skin & hair
- Fertility & menstruation
- Memory & concentration
- Bone strength
- Cholesterol level

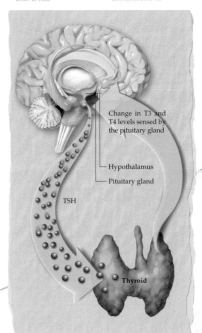

Normal Hormone Production

The thyroid gland is controlled by the pituitary gland. When the level of thyroid hormones (T3 & T4) drops too low, the pituitary gland responds by producing thyroid-stimulating hormone (TSH). TSH is a good marker of thyroid hormone balance: when the thyroid gland is underactive, TSH is high; when overactive, TSH is low.

Labels: Change in T3 and T4 levels sensed by the pituitary gland — Hypothalamus — Pituitary gland — TSH — Thyroid

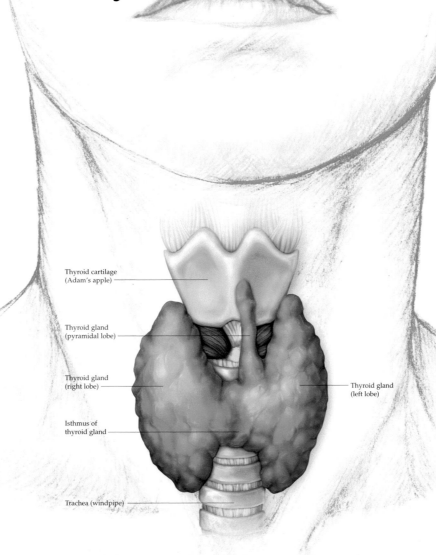

Labels: Thyroid cartilage (Adam's apple) — Thyroid gland (pyramidal lobe) — Thyroid gland (right lobe) — Thyroid gland (left lobe) — Isthmus of thyroid gland — Trachea (windpipe)

How to Check Your Thyroid

As a first step in identifying an underlying thyroid problem, you should do a simple thyroid self-exam.

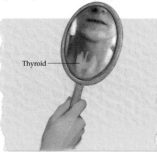

Label: Thyroid

1. While holding a mirror, look at the area of your neck just below the Adam's apple. This is where you will find your thyroid.

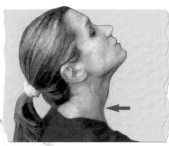

2. Tip your head back, while focusing on the thyroid area in the mirror.

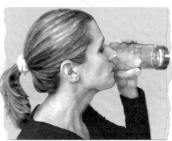

3. Take a drink of water. Look at your neck and check for any lumps in this area while you swallow.

Overactive Thyroid

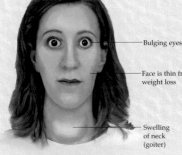

Broken lines indicate normal size of thyroid.

Labels: Bulging eyes — Face is thin from weight loss — Swelling of neck (goiter)

Common Thyroid Disorders

Overactive thyroid (hyperthyroidism):
When the thyroid gland is overactive, it makes too much of the thyroid hormone. This condition affects women more than men.

Graves' disease:
One of the most common causes of overactive thyroid, especially among women. It occurs when the immune system, which normally protects the body from bacteria and viruses, mistakenly attacks the thyroid gland and causes it to overproduce the thyroid hormone thyroxine. This autoimmune response can also affect the tissue behind the eyes (Graves' ophthalmopathy) and the skin on the shins (Graves' dermopathy).

Postpartum thyroiditis:
After childbirth, a woman's thyroid can become larger or inflamed. This condition usually goes away within six months, with no permanent damage to the thyroid.

Symptoms

- Sudden weight loss, even when appetite and food intake remain normal or increase.
- Rapid or irregular heartbeat or pounding of the heart.
- Nervousness, irritability, tremor.
- Sweating.
- Changes in menstrual patterns.
- Increased sensitivity to heat.
- Changes in bowel patterns, especially more frequent bowel movements.
- Enlarged thyroid (goiter), which may appear as a swelling at the base of the neck.
- Fatigue, muscle weakness.
- Difficulty sleeping.
- Pain or discomfort in the neck.

Underactive Thyroid

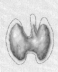

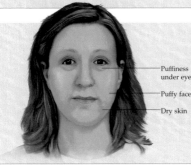

Broken lines indicate normal size of thyroid.

Labels: Puffiness under eyes — Puffy face — Dry skin

Underactive thyroid (hypothyroidism):
The most common type of thyroid disorder, where the thyroid makes too little of the thyroid hormone.

Hashimoto's disease:
The most often cause of underactive thyroid which can occur at any age but is most common in middle-aged and older women and in those who have a family history of this problem. It occurs when the immune system reacts against the thyroid gland, causing it to become inflamed (chronic thyroiditis).

Underactive thyroid and pregnancy:
A fetus depends on their mother's thyroid hormone for normal development. During pregnancy, women need more thyroid hormone, so thyroid testing is recommended every few weeks to ensure that the levels remain in balance.

- Increased sensitivity to cold.
- Constipation.
- Rough, cold, and dry skin.
- Puffy face.
- Hoarse voice.
- Poor concentration.
- Heavier-than-normal menstrual periods.
- Depression.
- Tingling sensations in legs and arms.
- Sleepiness.
- Unexplained weight gain.
Note: There may be no symptoms.

Thyroid Nodules and Cancer

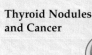

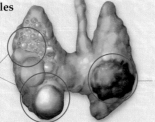

Labels: Nodules — Cancer

Thyroid nodules are extremely common and the vast majority are benign (not cancerous). Most commonly, nodules are discovered when a lump is noticed in the neck, or during an examination for another condition. Endocrinologists (thyroid specialists) often check to see if the nodule is not cancerous, and if surgery is recommended.

If **thyroid cancer** is found, it is usually highly treatable with an excellent prognosis. Surgical removal is usually the first step in treatment of thyroid cancer, sometimes followed by treatment with radioactive iodine.

- Lump in the front of the neck, on either side of the windpipe just below the Adam's apple.
- Tight feeling in the throat.
- Coughing.
- Hoarseness.
- Swollen lymph nodes, especially in the neck.
- Pain in the throat or neck, sometimes spreading up to the ears.

Other symptoms may occur depending on the cause of the lump(s).

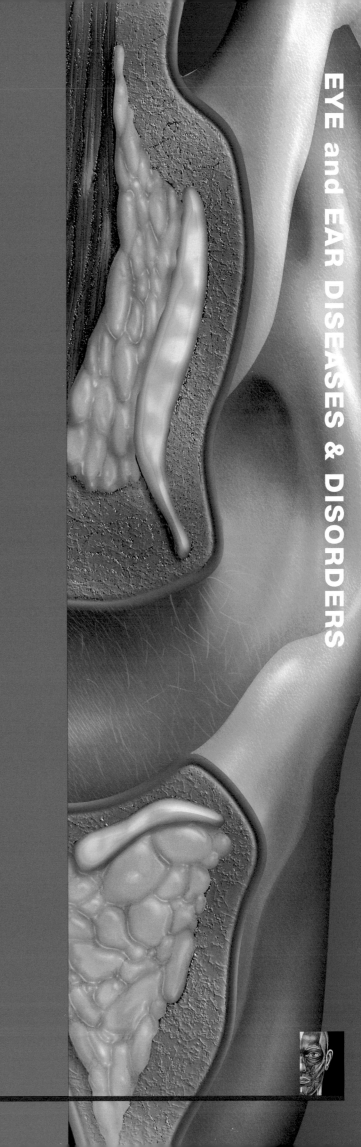

• Middle Ear Conditions • Disorders of the Eye • Understanding Glaucoma

Middle Ear Conditions

Otitis Media

Otitis media is an inflammation in the middle ear. It can be caused by bacteria, viruses, allergies, or malfunctions of the eustachian tube.

Inflammation may be accompanied by accumulation of fluid in the middle ear that may restrict the movement of the eardrum and middle ear ossicles, resulting in hearing loss. Pain may occur if there is pressure from fluid against the eardrum. Fever may result from an infection.

Normal Right Eardrum

Posterior superior quadrant
Anterior superior quadrant
Pars tensa
Umbo
Light reflex
Posterior inferior quadrant
Anterior inferior quadrant
Otoscope

Right auricle
Skull
External acoustic meatus
Lobule
Mastoid process
Epitympanum
Malleus
Incus
Stapes
Middle ear cavity
Tensor tympani muscle
Opening of eustachian tube to middle ear
Tympanic membrane (eardrum)
Isthmus
Osseous Portion
Cartilaginous Portion
Cartilage
Eustachian Tube
Levator veli palatini muscle
Styloid process

Middle Ear Development

Adult

Mastoid air cells
Aditus
Eustachian tube
Middle ear cavity
Infant

Dilator tubae
Eustachian tube
Tensor veli palatini muscle
Levator veli palatini muscle
Pterygoid hamulus

Nasal cavity
Opening of eustachian tube
Pharyngeal tonsil
Levator veli palatini muscle
Palatine Tonsil
Tongue

Drainage Tube Insertion

Myringotomy (Radial incision)
Front View
Side View
Drainage tube

Classification and Common Complications of Otitis Media

Acute Otitis Media†

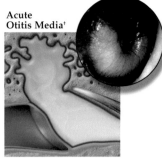

Infected fluid in the middle ear, of rapid onset and short duration.

Otitis Media with Effusion*

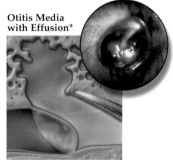

Relatively asymptomatic fluid in the middle ear that may be acute, subacute or chronic in nature.

Atelectasis

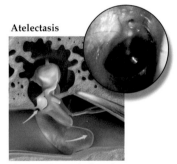

Thinning and potential collapse of the tympanic membrane.

Perforation*

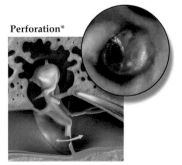

A hole in the tympanic membrane caused by chronic negative middle ear pressure, inflammation or trauma.

Cholesteatoma

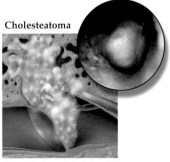

A mass of entrapped skin in the middle ear or temporal bone.

©2008 Wolters Kluwer Health | Lippincott Williams & Wilkins | Published by Anatomical Chart Company, Skokie, IL

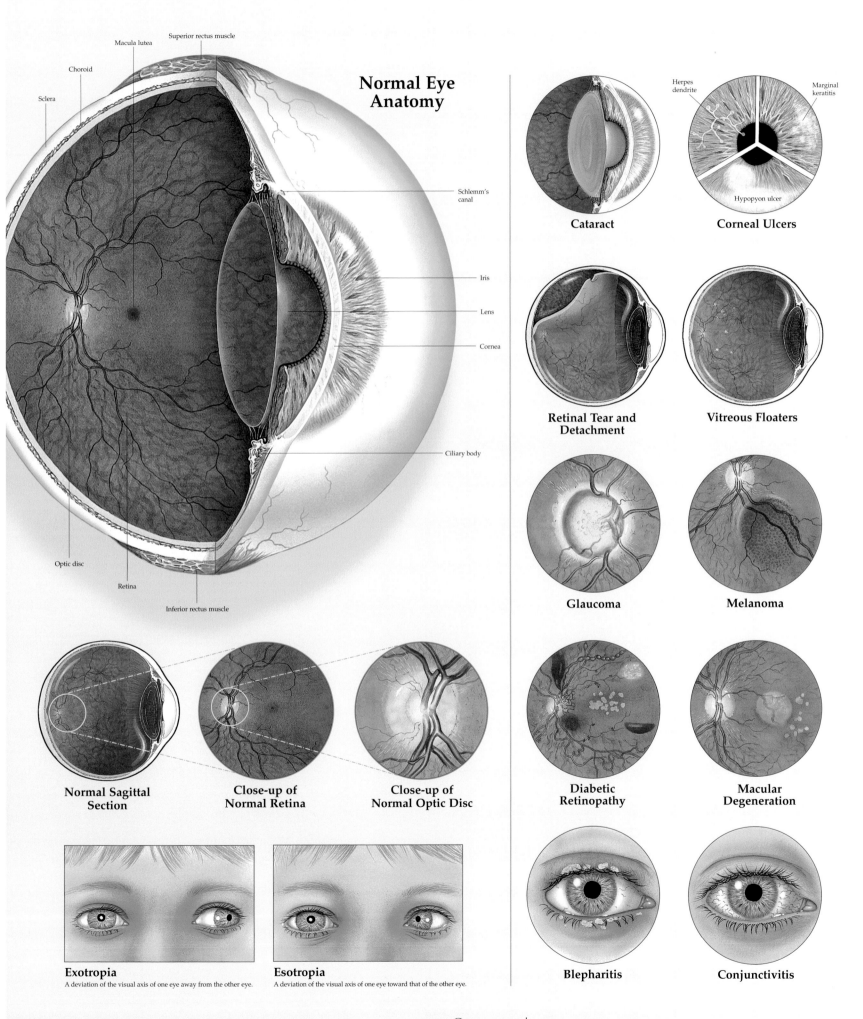

Normal Eye Anatomy

Superior rectus muscle

Macula lutea

Choroid

Sclera

Schlemm's canal

Iris

Lens

Cornea

Ciliary body

Optic disc

Retina

Inferior rectus muscle

Normal Sagittal Section

Close-up of Normal Retina

Close-up of Normal Optic Disc

Exotropia
A deviation of the visual axis of one eye away from the other eye.

Esotropia
A deviation of the visual axis of one eye toward that of the other eye.

Cataract

Corneal Ulcers

Herpes dendrite

Marginal keratitis

Hypopyon ulcer

Retinal Tear and Detachment

Vitreous Floaters

Glaucoma

Melanoma

Diabetic Retinopathy

Macular Degeneration

Blepharitis

Conjunctivitis

©2008 Wolters Kluwer Health | Lippincott Williams & Wilkins | Published by **Anatomical Chart Company, Skokie, IL**

Normal External Anatomy of the Left Eye

Caruncula

Lacrimal gland

Lacrimal punctum

Pupil   Iris   Sclera

Understanding Glaucoma

Glaucoma is a group of eye diseases that gradually steals sight without warning and often without symptoms. It is a condition in which normal fluid pressure inside the eyes (intraocular pressure, or IOP) slowly raises when the aqueous humor which normally flows in and out of the eye cannot drain properly. Instead, the fluid collects and causes pressure damage to the optic nerve (a bundle of more than 1 million nerve fibers that connect the retina with the brain) with subsequent loss of vision. There are sub-types of primary glaucoma: Open Angle, Narrow Angle, and Congenital.

Narrow Angle Glaucoma

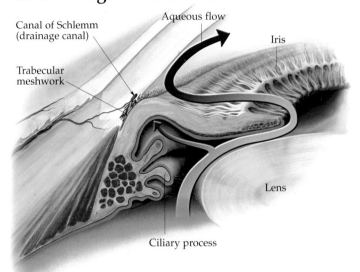

Aqueous flow

Canal of Schlemm (drainage canal)

Iris

Trabecular meshwork

Lens

Ciliary process

Narrow angle glaucoma, also known as closed angle glaucoma is much more rare and different from open angle glaucoma. Eye pressure usually goes up very fast. This happens when the drainage canal gets blocked or covered. The angle between the iris and the cornea is not as wide and open as it should be. Outer edges of the iris bunch up over the drainage canal when the pupil enlarges too much or too quickly.

Open Angle (Chronic) Glaucoma

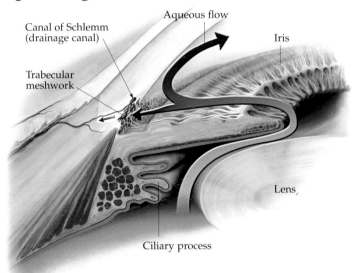

Aqueous flow

Canal of Schlemm (drainage canal)

Iris

Trabecular meshwork

Lens

Ciliary process

Open angle (chronic) glaucoma is the most common form of glaucoma. This happens when the aqueous fluid drainage canals (Canal of Schlemm) become constricted or obstructed over time. The inner eye pressure (intraocular pressure or IOP) rises because the correct amount of fluid cannot drain out of the eye. With open angle glaucoma, the entrances to the drainage canals are clear and should be working correctly. The obstruction occurs inside the drainage canals.

Congenital Glaucoma

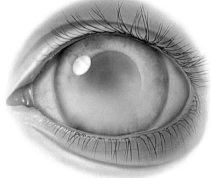

Congenital glaucoma is a rare form of glaucoma that occurs in babies and young children. This condition can be inherited. It is usually the result of incorrect or incomplete development of the eye's drainage canals during the prenatal period.

Sagittal View of the Eye

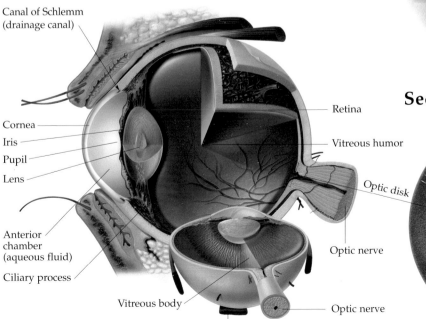

Canal of Schlemm (drainage canal)

Cornea

Iris

Pupil

Lens

Anterior chamber (aqueous fluid)

Ciliary process

Vitreous body

Inferior rectus muscle

Retina

Vitreous humor

Optic disk

Optic nerve

Optic nerve

Secondary Glaucoma

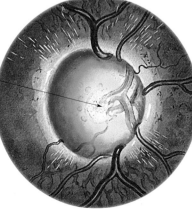

Secondary glaucoma can come from other medical conditions such as diabetes, eye surgery, advanced cataracts, eye injuries, certain eye tumors, eye infections, and eye inflammation. Certain drugs such as steroids can also be the cause and glaucoma may be mild or severe in diagnosis. Treatment includes medicines, laser surgery or conventional surgery.

©2008 Wolters Kluwer | Lippincott Williams & Wilkins | Published by Anatomical Chart Company, Skokie, IL
Health

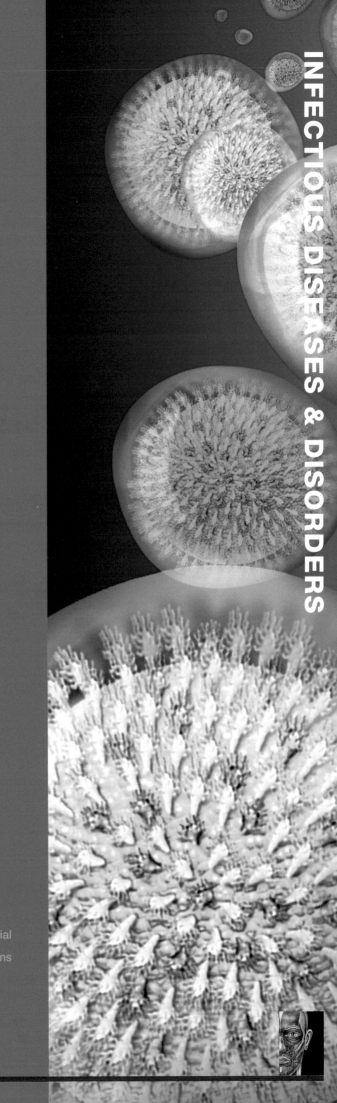

INFECTIOUS DISEASES & DISORDERS

• Understanding the Common Cold • Understanding Hepatitis • Understanding Bacterial Infections • Understanding HIV & AIDS • Understanding Influenza • Understanding Viral Infections

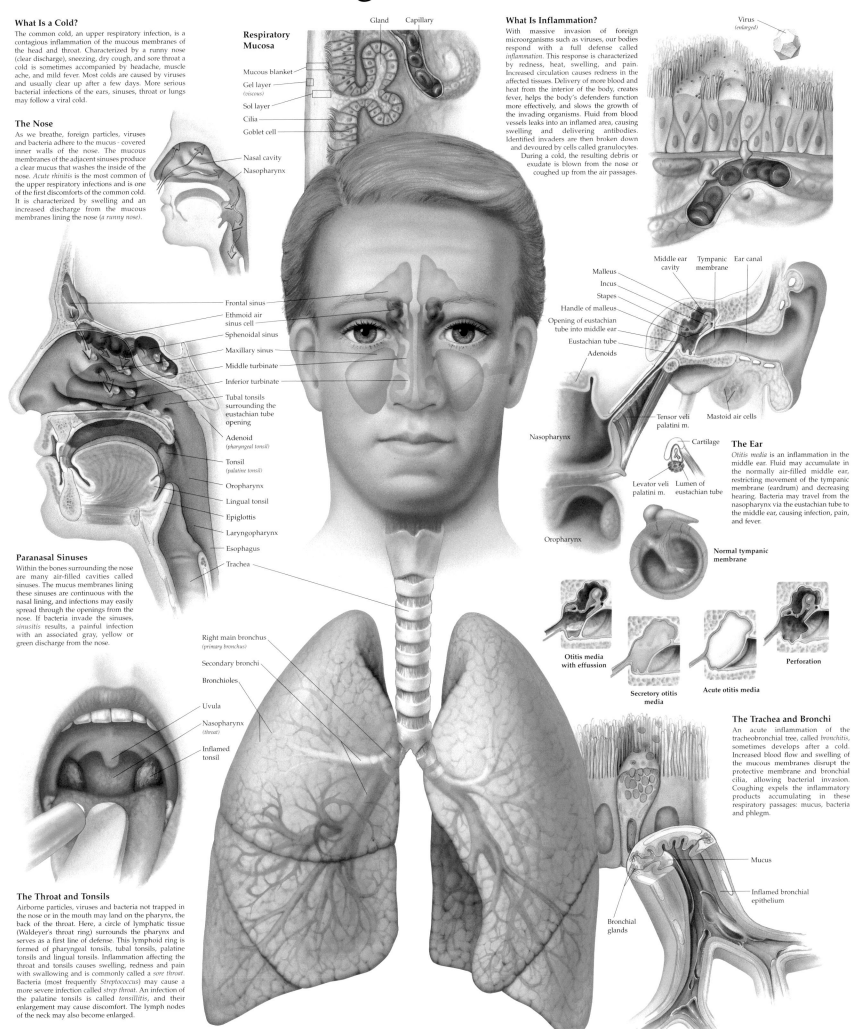

What Is a Cold?

The common cold, an upper respiratory infection, is a contagious inflammation of the mucous membranes of the head and throat. Characterized by a runny nose (clear discharge), sneezing, dry cough, and sore throat a cold is sometimes accompanied by headache, muscle ache, and mild fever. Most colds are caused by viruses and usually clear up after a few days. More serious bacterial infections of the ears, sinuses, throat or lungs may follow a viral cold.

The Nose

As we breathe, foreign particles, viruses and bacteria adhere to the mucus - covered inner walls of the nose. The mucous membranes of the adjacent sinuses produce a clear mucus that washes the inside of the nose. *Acute rhinitis* is the most common of the upper respiratory infections and is one of the first discomforts of the common cold. It is characterized by swelling and an increased discharge from the mucous membranes lining the nose (*a runny nose*).

Paranasal Sinuses

Within the bones surrounding the nose are many air-filled cavities called sinuses. The mucus membranes lining these sinuses are continuous with the nasal lining, and infections may easily spread through the openings from the nose. If bacteria invade the sinuses, *sinusitis* results, a painful infection with an associated gray, yellow or green discharge from the nose.

The Throat and Tonsils

Airborne particles, viruses and bacteria not trapped in the nose or in the mouth may land on the pharynx, the back of the throat. Here, a circle of lymphatic tissue (Waldeyer's throat ring) surrounds the pharynx and serves as a first line of defense. This lymphoid ring is formed of pharyngeal tonsils, tubal tonsils, palatine tonsils and lingual tonsils. Inflammation affecting the throat and tonsils causes swelling, redness and pain with swallowing and is commonly called a *sore throat*. Bacteria (most frequently *Streptococcus*) may cause a more severe infection called *strep throat*. An infection of the palatine tonsils is called *tonsillitis*, and their enlargement may cause discomfort. The lymph nodes of the neck may also become enlarged.

Respiratory Mucosa

Gland
Capillary
Mucous blanket
Gel layer (viscous)
Sol layer
Cilia
Goblet cell
Nasal cavity
Nasopharynx

Frontal sinus
Ethmoid air sinus cell
Sphenoidal sinus
Maxillary sinus
Middle turbinate
Inferior turbinate
Tubal tonsils surrounding the eustachian tube opening
Adenoid (pharyngeal tonsil)
Tonsil (palatine tonsil)
Oropharynx
Lingual tonsil
Epiglottis
Laryngopharynx
Esophagus
Trachea

Right main bronchus (primary bronchus)
Secondary bronchi
Bronchioles
Uvula
Nasopharynx (throat)
Inflamed tonsil

What Is Inflammation?

With massive invasion of foreign microorganisms such as viruses, our bodies respond with a full defense called *inflammation*. This response is characterized by redness, heat, swelling, and pain. Increased circulation causes redness in the affected tissues. Delivery of more blood and heat from the interior of the body, creates fever, helps the body's defenders function more effectively, and slows the growth of the invading organisms. Fluid from blood vessels leaks into an inflamed area, causing swelling and delivering antibodies. Identified invaders are then broken down and devoured by cells called granulocytes. During a cold, the resulting debris or exudate is blown from the nose or coughed up from the air passages.

Virus (enlarged)

Middle ear cavity
Tympanic membrane
Ear canal
Malleus
Incus
Stapes
Handle of malleus
Opening of eustachian tube into middle ear
Eustachian tube
Adenoids
Tensor veli palatini m.
Mastoid air cells
Nasopharynx
Cartilage
Levator veli palatini m.
Lumen of eustachian tube
Oropharynx

The Ear

Otitis media is an inflammation in the middle ear. Fluid may accumulate in the normally air-filled middle ear, restricting movement of the tympanic membrane (eardrum) and decreasing hearing. Bacteria may travel from the nasopharynx via the eustachian tube to the middle ear, causing infection, pain, and fever.

Normal tympanic membrane

Otitis media with effussion
Secretory otitis media
Acute otitis media
Perforation

The Trachea and Bronchi

An acute inflammation of the tracheobronchial tree, called *bronchitis*, sometimes develops after a cold. Increased blood flow and swelling of the mucous membranes disrupt the protective membrane and bronchial cilia, allowing bacterial invasion. Coughing expels the inflammatory products accumulating in these respiratory passages: mucus, bacteria and phlegm.

Mucus
Inflamed bronchial epithelium
Bronchial glands

©2008 Wolters Kluwer | Lippincott Williams & Wilkins | Published by Anatomical Chart Company, Skokie, IL

Understanding Hepatitis

What is Viral Hepatitis?

Viral hepatitis is a fairly common disease leading to the destruction of liver cells. It is caused by one or more of five different hepatic viruses (Hepatitis A, B, C, D and E) some singly, some in combination. The disease progresses from the preicteric (before the onset of jaundice) period, through the icteric period, and finally to the posticteric period. While most people are asymptomatic and recover completely, others develop chronic hepatitis. People at increased risk for hepatitis include intravenous drug users, health care workers, infants born to infected mothers, hemodialysis patients, recipients of plasma-derived products, travelers from areas where hepatitis is endemic, and people who have multiple sexual partners.

Transmission of Hepatitis

Hepatitis A and E are spread by the consumption of fecally contaminated food, milk or water. Hepatitis B, C, and D are spread by exposure to blood/blood products or secretions of an infected person, and at birth by an infected mother to her infant.

Complications of Hepatitis

Chronic hepatitis can lead to cirrhosis and even liver cancer. Cirrhosis causes the liver to begin to shrink and harden. Scarring of the liver can also occur, which can lead to permanent impairment of liver function.

Cirrhosis

As cirrhosis progresses, other detrimental changes can take place. **Portal hypertension** is induced by an increased resistance to blood flow through the liver. Limited blood flow through the liver causes splanchnic arterial flow to increase at the same time. These two factors when combined can overload the portal system. Increased pressure stimulates the development of collateral channels (**varices**), which attempt to bypass the portal vein flow into the liver. Portal hypertension causes **splenomegaly** (enlargement of the spleen), **ascites** (fluid retention in the abdomen), blood clotting deficiencies, and **hepatic encephalopathy** (mental confusion). In addition, the liver can lose its ability to remove waste products from the blood.

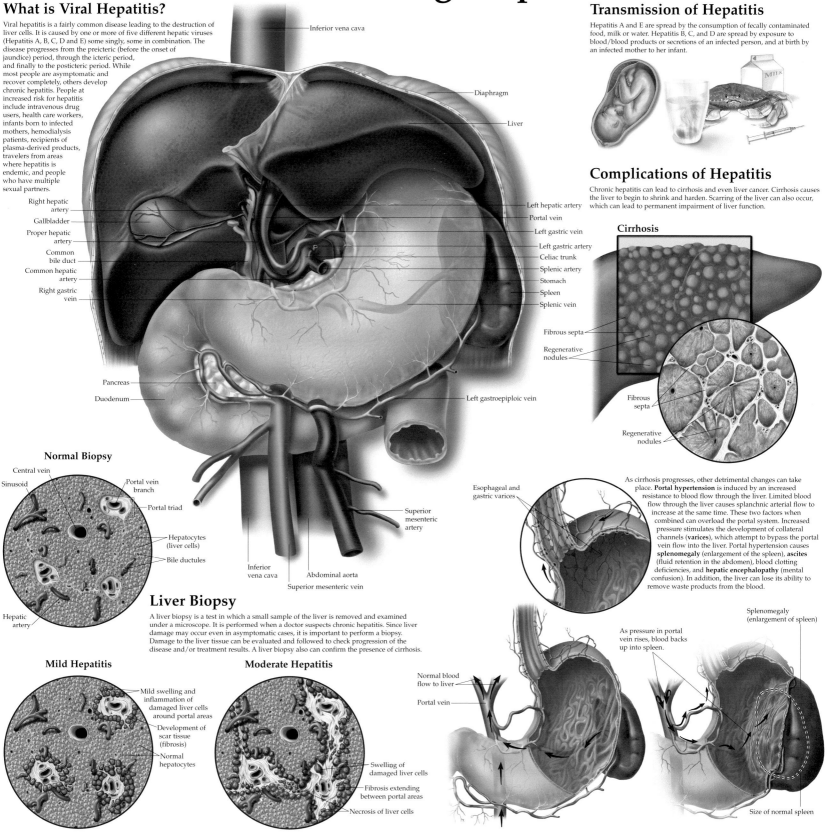

Labels: Inferior vena cava; Diaphragm; Liver; Right hepatic artery; Gallbladder; Proper hepatic artery; Common bile duct; Common hepatic artery; Right gastric vein; Pancreas; Duodenum; Left hepatic artery; Portal vein; Left gastric vein; Left gastric artery; Celiac trunk; Splenic artery; Stomach; Spleen; Splenic vein; Left gastroepiploic vein; Superior mesenteric artery; Inferior vena cava; Abdominal aorta; Superior mesenteric vein

Normal Biopsy
Labels: Central vein; Sinusoid; Portal vein branch; Portal triad; Hepatocytes (liver cells); Bile ductules; Hepatic artery

Cirrhosis (micrograph)
Labels: Fibrous septa; Regenerative nodules; Fibrous septa; Regenerative nodules

Labels: Esophageal and gastric varices; Normal blood flow to liver; Portal vein; As pressure in portal vein rises, blood backs up into spleen; Splenomegaly (enlargement of spleen); Size of normal spleen

Liver Biopsy

A liver biopsy is a test in which a small sample of the liver is removed and examined under a microscope. It is performed when a doctor suspects chronic hepatitis. Since liver damage may occur even in asymptomatic cases, it is important to perform a biopsy. Damage to the liver tissue can be evaluated and followed to check progression of the disease and/or treatment results. A liver biopsy also can confirm the presence of cirrhosis.

Mild Hepatitis
Labels: Mild swelling and inflammation of damaged liver cells around portal areas; Development of scar tissue (fibrosis); Normal hepatocytes

Moderate Hepatitis
Labels: Swelling of damaged liver cells; Fibrosis extending between portal areas; Necrosis of liver cells

Types of Hepatitis

- **Hepatitis A Virus (HAV)**
  HAV is the most prevalent form of hepatitis in the United States and is very contagious. It is spread by the ingestion of fecally contaminated foods or water. Transmission by exposure to contaminated blood is rare.

- **Hepatitis B Virus (HBV)**
  HBV is spread by contact with secretions, feces or blood of an infected person. It is also transmitted by sexual contact and during birth. Hepatitis B is a particular risk for health care workers and is increasing among HIV-positive patients. HBV can result in cirrhosis and liver cancer.

- **Hepatitis C Virus (HCV)**
  HCV is transmitted by blood transfusion from an infected donor, by sexual contact with an infected person, and from mother to child at birth. The hepatitis C virus can produce chronic infection, chronic liver disease, cirrhosis, and liver cancer.

- **Hepatitis D Virus (HDV)**
  HDV occurs only in those infected with the hepatitis B virus. It causes cirrhosis as well as sudden, severe illness that can be fatal. It is usually transmitted by contact with contaminated blood.

- **Hepatitis E Virus (HEV)**
  HEV occurs primarily in those who have traveled to developing countries. It is transmitted by the consumption of fecally contaminated food or water.

- **Hepatitis G Virus (HGV) and Transfusion Transmitted Virus (TTV)**
  HGV and TTV are recently discovered viruses. So far, these viruses do not appear to be associated with clinical hepatitis or any liver injury. Research is being conducted to provide more information about these viruses.

Signs and Symptoms

All types of hepatitis present similar symptoms, which progress in the following three stages:

- **Prodromal or preicteric stage**
  Initially, a patient with hepatitis may exhibit flu-like symptoms, such as low-grade fever, loss of appetite, nausea, vomiting, fatigue, muscle and joint pain, headache, general discomfort, and cough. This stage may last from twelve to fourteen days.

- **Clinical jaundice or icteric stage**
  Some patients develop jaundice, which is a result of damaged liver cells, impaired liver function, and the accumulation of the pigment bilirubin in the blood. One to five days prior to jaundice, there may be mild weight loss, yellow eyes and skin, dark urine, and light-colored stool. After the onset of jaundice, the liver enlarges and becomes tender. The spleen may also become enlarged. This stage lasts from one to two weeks.

- **Recovery or posticteric stage**
  Most symptoms abate or disappear. There is also a decrease in the size of the liver. This stage lasts from two to twelve weeks, often longer in patients with hepatitis B, C, or E.

Understanding Bacterial Infections

46

Basic Structure of Bacteria

- Flagellum
- Capsule
- Cell wall
- Cell membrane
- Nucleoid
- Cytoplasm

BACTERIAL INFECTIONS

Pathogenic *(disease-producing)* bacteria may enter the body through the mouth, nose, and cuts or bites on the skin. Once inside the body, the bacteria may multiply sufficiently to cause illness. Illnesses caused by bacteria and other microorganisms are called infections. Infections may be caused directly by the bacteria or by their poisonous waste products, called *toxins*.

Three Ways Bacteria Cause Damage

1 Tissue Damage
Some bacteria may adhere to and invade tissue cells. Other bacteria may produce toxins that alter the chemical reactions in cells. This results in a disruption in the cells' normal function or causes the cell to die.

- Toxins
- Bacteria
- Damaged tissue

- Bacteria
- Red blood cell
- Toxins
- Fibrin *(involved with clotting)*
- Blood vessel

2 Blood Clots *(intravascular coagulation)*
Some bacterial toxins may cause blood to coagulate *(clot)* in small vessels, forming blockages. The tissue cells normally supplied by these vessels are deprived of blood, resulting in tissue damage.

3 Fluid Leakage from Vessel
The walls of small blood vessels may be damaged by bacterial toxins. This leads to fluid leakage from the vessel into the surrounding tissue. The fluid loss results in decreased blood pressure, and the heart is unable to pump an adequate amount of blood to the vital organs.

- Damaged vessel wall
- Bacteria
- Toxin

- Fluid leakage

Pathogenic Bacteria

Neisseria meningitidis
- *Types of infection:*
- Meningitis

Streptococcus pyogenes
- Septicemia
- Myositis
- Necrotizing fasciitis

Streptococcus pneumoniae
- Pneumonia
- Meningitis
- Otitis media

Staphylococcus aureus
- Endocarditis
- Cellulitis
- Pneumonia
- Osteomyelitis
- Septicemia

Escherichia coli
- Urogenital tract infection
- Diarrhea

Salmonella typhi
- Enterocolitis
- Bacteremia
- Typhoid
- Localized infections

Pseudomonas aeruginosa
- Urinary infection
- Wound infection

Sites of Infection

Key
A - Brain
B - Lung
C - Heart
D - Liver
E - Stomach
F - Large intestine
G - Small intestine
H - Bladder

BACTERIAL INFECTIONS MAY LEAD TO SEPSIS

What Is Sepsis?

Sepsis is a systemic inflammatory response syndrome resulting from a **bacterial infection**. In sepsis, bacteria from the infected site, or the toxins they produce, enter the bloodstream and spread throughout the body. This sets off a chain of chemical reactions that lead to excessive systemic inflammation and intravascular coagulation. Without proper treatment, this may lead to organ dysfunction, multiple organ failure, and eventually death.

What Are the Risk Factors?

People with inefficient immune systems or blood disorders are at particular risk for sepsis. The risk factors associated with sepsis include:

- Major surgery
- Chemotherapy
- Immunosuppressive medications
- Therapy with antibiotics
- Indwelling catheters/tubes
- An endoscopic procedure
- A cardiovascular procedure

What Are the Causes of Sepsis?

Sepsis is a result of a bacterial infection that can originate anywhere in the body. **Sites of infection** may include the lungs, digestive tract, kidneys, bladder, joints, skin, or the coverings around the brain.
Infections that can cause sepsis include:

- Meningitis *(inflammation of the brain membrane)*
- Bacterial pneumonia *(inflammation of the lungs)*
- Bacterial peritonitis *(inflammation of the peritoneum)*
- Osteomyelitis *(infection of the cortical bone)*
- Septic arthritis *(inflammation of synovial membrane of joints)*
- Cellulitis *(inflammation of subcutaneous, connective tissue)*
- Endocarditis *(infection of the valves of the heart)*
- Bacterial enterocolitis *(infection of the small and large intestines)*
- Cholecystitis *(inflammation of the gallbladder)*
- Ascending cholangitis *(inflammation of bile duct or biliary tree)*
- Pyelonephritis *(inflammation of the kidney)*
- Cystitis *(inflammation of the urinary bladder)*

What Are the Symptoms?

Symptoms of sepsis include:

- High fever
- Low body temperature
- Chills with body shaking
- Confusion or changes in mental status
- Hyperventilation *(rapid breathing)*
- Tachycardia *(rapid heartbeat)*
- Low urine production

What Are the Complications?

When an infection worsens, bacteria may enter the bloodstream. Toxins produced by the bacteria can affect the blood vessels by causing **intravascular coagulation** or **fluid leakage** from the vessel. The result is severe hypotension *(low blood pressure)*, which is known as *septic shock*. Impaired blood flow can result in damage to vital organs such as the brain, heart, and kidneys.

What Is the Treatment?

Hospitalization is necessary to treat sepsis successfully. Blood culture tests are performed to identify the causative **pathogenic bacteria**. While the test results are pending, intravenous antibiotic therapy is administered to the patient. This consists of a broad-spectrum *(kills a variety of bacteria)* antibiotic or multiple antibiotics. When the test results become available, the treatment can then be tailored to combat the causative pathogenic bacteria. Further testing may be done to identify the source or originating **site of the infection**. Supportive therapy with oxygen, intravenous fluids, and medications to restore normal blood pressure, is also important for a complete recovery.

©2008 Wolters Kluwer | Lippincott Williams & Wilkins | Published by Anatomical Chart Company, Skokie, IL
Health

Understanding HIV and AIDS

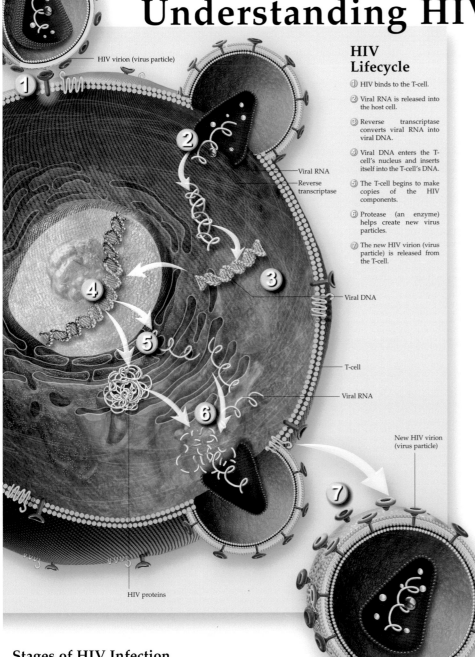

47

HIV virion (virus particle)

1

2

Viral RNA

Reverse transcriptase

4

5

Viral DNA

T-cell

Viral RNA

6

New HIV virion (virus particle)

7

HIV proteins

HIV Lifecycle

① HIV binds to the T-cell.

② Viral RNA is released into the host cell.

③ Reverse transcriptase converts viral RNA into viral DNA.

④ Viral DNA enters the T-cell's nucleus and inserts itself into the T-cell's DNA.

⑤ The T-cell begins to make copies of the HIV components.

⑥ Protease (an enzyme) helps create new virus particles.

⑦ The new HIV virion (virus particle) is released from the T-cell.

What Are HIV and AIDS?

Since it was first reported in 1981, HIV/AIDs has become a major worldwide epidemic. AIDS (acquired immunodeficiency syndrome) is a chronic, life-threatening condition caused by the human immunodeficiency virus (HIV). HIV damages or destroys certain cells of the immune system, particularly T-cells, weakening the body's response to infections and certain types of cancers. The virus and the infection are known as HIV, while the term "AIDS" refers to the later stages of HIV infection.

HIV Testing

HIV tests tell patients if they are infected with the human immunodeficiency virus (HIV). The tests look for antibodies (proteins made by the immune system to fight a specific disease) to HIV. The most common type of HIV test is a blood test known as an enzyme-linked immunosorbent assay (ELISA) screening. It searches for antibodies to HIV in the blood. A positive result should always be confirmed with a second test. Another blood test is called the Western blot analysis, which looks for antibodies to several HIV proteins.

How Is HIV Transmitted?

Sexual Activity
Having unprotected sexual contact with an infected partner is the most common method of spreading HIV. Contact with infected blood, semen, or vaginal secretions can lead to the transmission of HIV.

Pregnancy
A woman can transmit the virus to her unborn infant during pregnancy, delivery, or after birth when she is breastfeeding. Babies born to infected mothers have a 15% to 25% chance of becoming infected.

Contaminated Needles
The virus can survive for several days in the small amounts of blood left in a needle after use. Used needles are a high risk for HIV transmission. Injection needles can pass blood directly from one person's bloodstream to another.

Blood or Blood Products
Infected blood is where HIV is found in the highest concentrations. Since 1985 the HIV antibody test has been used to screen blood donations for the virus. Now it is rare to become infected by receiving blood or blood products through transfusion.

HIV is **not** transmitted by insect bites; casual contact; sharing dishes or food; swimming pools and hot tubs; pets; contact with saliva, tears, or sweat; contact with toilets; or donating blood.

Risk Factors

Anyone of any age, race, gender, or sexual orientation can become infected with HIV, but a person is at greatest risk if he or she:

• Has unprotected sex with multiple partners.

• Has unprotected sex with a partner who is HIV-positive.

• Has another sexually transmitted infection such as syphilis, herpes, or gonorrhea.

• Shares needles during intravenous drug use.

• Is a hemophiliac who received blood products before April 1985.

• Received a blood transfusion or blood products before 1985.

Newborns or nursing infants whose mothers are HIV-positive are also at high risk. Anyone at risk should be tested for HIV infection.

AIDS-Related Illnesses

Opportunistic infections (OIs) occur only when the immune system is severely damaged. These infections cause life-threatening illnesses in people with AIDS. Below is a partial list of some of the infections/cancers associated with AIDS, along with some of their symptoms.

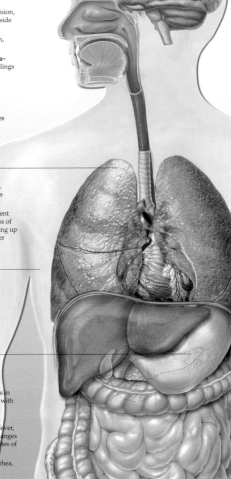

Nervous system:

• Toxoplasmosis– fever, headache, partial loss of vision, seizures, paralysis on one side of the body, confusion

• Cryptococcosis– confusion, fever, headache, seizures

• Non-Hodgkin's lymphoma– one or more painless swellings in neck, armpits, or groin; fever, sweats

• Herpes zoster (shingles)– painful rash of fluid-filled blisters found on chest, abdomen, face or extremities

Respiratory system:

• Pneumocystis carinii pneumoni (PCP)– fatigue, fever, dry cough, shortness of breath

• Tuberculosis (TB)– persistent cough, chest pain, shortness of breath, weight loss, coughing up of blood (hemoptysis), fever

Skin:

• Herpes simplex– painful blisters on or around lips or genitals

• Kaposi's sarcoma– raised, purple or pinkish-brown lesions on skin

Digestive system:

• Cryptosporidiosis– watery diarrhea, abdominal pain, fever, vomiting

• Candidiasis– white plaques in mouth and/or throat, pain with swallowing or eating

• Cytomegalovirus (CMV)– diarrhea, non-itchy rash, fever, abdominal pain, visual changes yellowing of skin and whites of eyes (very rare)

• Isosporiasis– watery diarrhea, abdominal pain, weight loss, fever

Stages of HIV Infection

1. Acute Stage
Occurs about 1 to 2 weeks after initial infection. During this stage, the virus undergoes massive replication. Patients may be asymptomatic or have a flu-like syndrome.

2. Asymptomatic HIV
During this stage, chronic signs or symptoms are not present. T-cell count may be used to monitor progression of the disease. With the patient's own resistance and drug therapy, this stage can last for 10 to 12 years or longer.

3. Symptomatic HIV
This stage has two phases: early and late. When the T-cell count falls below 200 cells per cubic millimeter of blood, it is the late phase. This stage of HIV is defined mainly by the emergence of opportunistic infections and cancers to which the immune system normally helps maintain resistance.

4. Advanced HIV
A T-cell count of 50 cells per cubic millimeter or less represents advanced HIV. With the onset of this stage, patients are at the highest risk for opportunistic infections and malignancies.

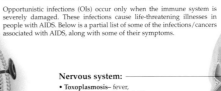

Acute Stage | Asymptomatic HIV | Symptomatic HIV | Advanced HIV

T-cells (CD4)/ mm^3
1200 / 1100 / 1000 / 900 / 800 / 700 / 600 / 500 / 400 / 300 / 200 / 100 / 0

HIV RNA Copies per ml Plasma
10^7 / 10^6 / 10^5 / 10^4 / 10^3 / 10^2

T-cells

HIV RNA

Weeks: 0 3 6 9 12
Years: 1 2 3 4 5 6 7 8 9 10 11

Signs and Symptoms of HIV Infection

Depending on the stage of infection, the symptoms of HIV vary. Symptoms can include:

• Short-term memory loss
• Persistent headaches
• High fever
• Confusion and forgetfulness
• Seizures and lack of coordination

• Persistent or frequent oral infections
• Difficult or painful swallowing
• Loss of appetite
• Heavy night sweats
• Cough and shortness of breath

• Swollen lymph nodes in neck, armpits, and groin
• Persistent skin rashes or flaky skin
• Severe weight loss
• Chronic diarrhea
• Lack of energy and muscle weakness

Treatment

HIV and AIDS are not curable, but early detection and treatment can increase life expectancy. There are no vaccines available, but medications can slow the progression of HIV and the development of AIDS. Other medications are available to protect against and treat the variety of illnesses that may develop. Consult with a physician that specializes in caring for HIV-infected individuals. It is critical that all prescribed medication be taken as directed.

Understanding Influenza

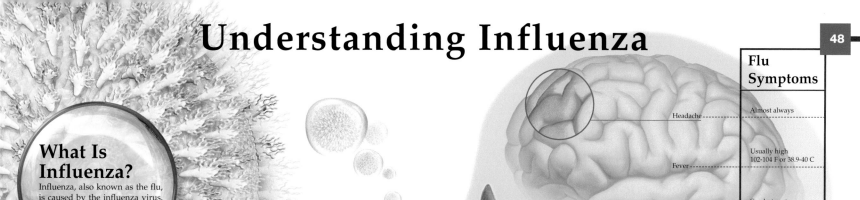

Flu Symptoms

Headache	Almost always
Fever	Usually high 102-104 F or 38.9-40 C
Fatigue, weakness	Can last up to two to three weeks
Runny or stuffy nose	Sometimes
Sneezing	Sometimes
Sore throat	Sometimes
Cough	Can become severe
Chest discomfort	Common
General aches, pains	Usually, often severe

What Is Influenza?

Influenza, also known as the flu, is caused by the influenza virus. It is a contagious infection of the nose, throat, and lungs.

Influenza virus spreads in the little drops that spray out of an infected person's mouth and nose when he sneezes, coughs, laughs, or even talks.

When someone else breathes in these drops or gets them on his hands and then touches his own mouth or nose, the virus can enter his body .

Prevention

Ways to Help Prevent Influenza

Avoid touching your eyes, nose, and mouth.

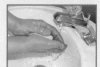

Wash your hands with soap and water frequently.

Get a vaccination (flu shot) every year before the start of the flu season. *Note: The vaccine does not cause the flu.*

Ways to Help Prevent the Spread of Influenza

Stay home when you are sick.

Avoid close contact with others.

Cover your mouth and nose with a tissue when coughing or sneezing.

Special Risk Factors

Certain people have an increased risk of serious complications from influenza:
• People age 65 years and older
• People of any age with chronic medical conditions
• Pregnant women
• Children between 6 months and 23 months of age

Flu Vaccination (Flu Shot)

Because the influenza virus is different every year, you should protect yourself by getting a flu shot every year. If you are at high risk for major complications from the flu, it is especially important to get the shot before the flu season. The influenza vaccine may also lessen the severity of symptoms related to other forms of influenza that the vaccine is unable to prevent. The flu shot will not protect you from the common cold.

Complications

The complications caused by influenza include:
• Bacterial pneumonia
• Dehydration
• Worsening of chronic medical conditions, such as congestive heart failure, asthma, or diabetes
• Children may develop sinus problems or ear infections

Most people who get influenza recover in one to two weeks, but some people develop life-threatening complications (such as pneumonia) as a result of the flu. If your flu symptoms are unusually severe , you should seek medical help immediately.

Bronchitis, or inflammation of the bronchi, is another complication of influenza. In most cases, it involves the large and medium-sized bronchi. In children, older people, and those with lung disease, the infection may spread and inflame the bronchioles or lung tissue.

Bronchitis

What to Do If You Get Sick

If you develop an influenza infection, you should:
• Get plenty of rest
• Drink plenty of liquids
• Avoid using alcohol and tobacco

You can also take medications to relieve flu symptoms but never give aspirin to children or teenagers who have cold or flu symptoms without first speaking to your healthcare provider. Antiviral medications have been approved for treatment of influenza but must be prescribed by a doctor. There is no cure for the flu. The antiviral medications can help reduce the severity and the duration of the symptoms.

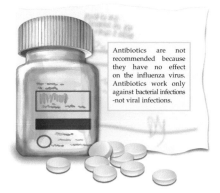

Antibiotics are not recommended because they have no effect on the influenza virus. Antibiotics work only against bacterial infections -not viral infections.

Questions & Answers

Q: How can you tell the difference between a common cold and influenza ?

A: Although flu and cold symptoms can be similar, the intensity and duration are different. The symptoms of a cold may come on gradually and are milder than the symptoms of the flu. Flu symptoms are more severe and tend to come on immediately and take longer to recover.

Q: Is the stomach flu the same type of flu as influenza (flu)?

A: No. Some people use the term "stomach flu" to describe certain common illnesses that can cause nausea, vomiting, or diarrhea. Although these symptoms can sometimes be related to the flu (more commonly in children), these problems are rarely symptoms of influenza.

Q: Can the symptoms of influenza (flu) be different in children?

A: Yes. Although flu symptoms for children and adults might be similar, children might have other symptoms such as nausea, vomiting and/or diarrhea. Children are at a higher risk of complications from the flu. If a child's symptoms worsen, call your doctor.

©2008 Wolters Kluwer Health | Lippincott Williams & Wilkins | Published by Anatomical Chart Company, Skokie, IL

B How Viruses Infect Cells

A virus is unable to process nutrients or replicate without a host cell.

1 To invade a cell, the surface proteins on the virus attach to specific receptor sites on the host cell's outer membrane.

2 After attaching to the membrane, part or all of the virus penetrates into the host cell.

3 Depending on the specific virus, the nucleic acid of the virus is released into the host cell's cytoplasm or nucleus. Then the viral genes direct the production of proteins and nucleic acids, the components of new virus particles.

4 The host cells may burst, releasing the viruses to infect other cells. However, not all viruses destroy the cell as they leave. Some viruses form buds from the host cell's membrane and are released.

C Viral Entry Sites

Eye / conjunctiva

Mouth / oropharynx

Skin

Respiratory tract

Intestinal tract

Urogenital tract

Key
a - Brain
b - Lung
c - Heart
d - Liver
e - Stomach
f - Large intestine
g - Small intestine
h - Bladder

A General Structure of a Virus

Double lipid layer

Nucleic acid
(Composed of DNA or RNA)

Protein shell

Surface protein
(Antigen)

D Viral Spread via the Blood

Viremia is the presence of a virus in the bloodstream. Blood-borne viruses either circulate freely in the plasma or are cell-associated. Cell-associated viremia means that the virus replicates in cells found in the circulation, particularly B or T lymphocytes or monocytes, or *(rarely)* red blood cells.

Monocyte
(White blood cell)

Red blood cell

Cell-associated viremia

Plasma viremia

Blood vessel

What Is a Virus?

Viruses are subcellular organisms made up of RNA *(ribonucleic acid)* or DNA *(deoxyribonucleic acid)* covered with proteins. Viruses are obligate intracellular parasites, meaning that they are incapable of growth or reproduction apart from living cells. Instead, they invade a host cell and stimulate it to participate in the formation of additional virus particles. Viruses are classified according to their size, shape *(spherical, rod-shaped, or cubic)*, or means of transmission *(respiratory, fecal, oral, or sexual)*.

A General Structure of a Virus

A virus has a core of nucleic acid, composed of DNA or RNA, depending on what type of virus it is. The nucleic acid is enclosed in one or two protein shells. Surface proteins *(antigens)* cover the outer shell.

B How Viruses Infect Cells

Viruses invade host cells by attaching to a specific molecule on the cell surface, which acts as a receptor. Following attachment, there is a multi-step entry process that delivers the viral nucleic acid, which contains the genes, into either the cytoplasm or the nucleus of the host cell. Once released, the viral genes dictate the synthesis of viral proteins and the replication of its genome, followed by assembly and release of new virus particles. Cell destruction is required for release of some viruses but not of others, which "bud" through the plasma membrane.

What Are the Modes of Transmission?

Most infectious diseases are transmitted in one of four ways.

1. In **contact transmission**, the susceptible host comes into direct contact *(as in sexually transmitted disease)* or indirect contact *(contaminated inanimate objects)* with the source.
2. **Airborne transmission** results from inhalation of contaminated fine mist droplets, which are sometimes suspended in airborne dust particles.
3. In **enteric** *(oral-fecal)* **transmission**, the infecting organisms are found in feces and are ingested by susceptible hosts, either by direct contact or, in some cases, through fecally contaminated food or water.
4. **Vector-borne transmission** occurs when an intermediate carrier *(vector)*, such as a flea or a mosquito, transfers an organism.

C Viral Entry Sites

The first step of infection is entry into the host. This can occur at the following sites:

- Conjunctiva *(mucous membranes of the eye)*
- Mouth / oropharynx
- Skin
- Respiratory tract
- Intestinal tract
- Urogenital tract

How Viruses Spread in the Body

Some viruses are confined to the site of initial infection and spread only locally, whereas others spread widely. In the body, viruses may spread via the blood or via the peripheral nervous system.

D Viral Spread Via the Blood

Viremia is the presence of a virus in the bloodstream. The most common source of viremia is a virus that replicates in regional lymph nodes and is transported by the thoracic duct into the circulation. Blood-borne viruses either circulate freely in the plasma or are cell-associated. Most viremias are acute, lasting no more than one to two weeks. However, certain viruses are able to evade immune defenses and persist in the blood for months or years. Human immunodeficiency virus, the cause of AIDS, is an example of a persistent viremia. Blood-borne viruses can invade almost any organ or cell type.

Viral Spread Via the Peripheral Nervous System

Neural spread is a process by which a virus is transmitted within the axon of peripheral nerve fibers. The neural pathway plays an essential role in the spread of some viruses, although it is less common than viremia as a mode of spread. Neurotropic viruses are usually confined to the peripheral and central nervous systems and replicate in relatively few peripheral tissues. Rabies virus is an example of a neurotropic virus.

©2008 Wolters Kluwer Health | Lippincott Williams & Wilkins | Published by Anatomical Chart Company, Skokie, IL

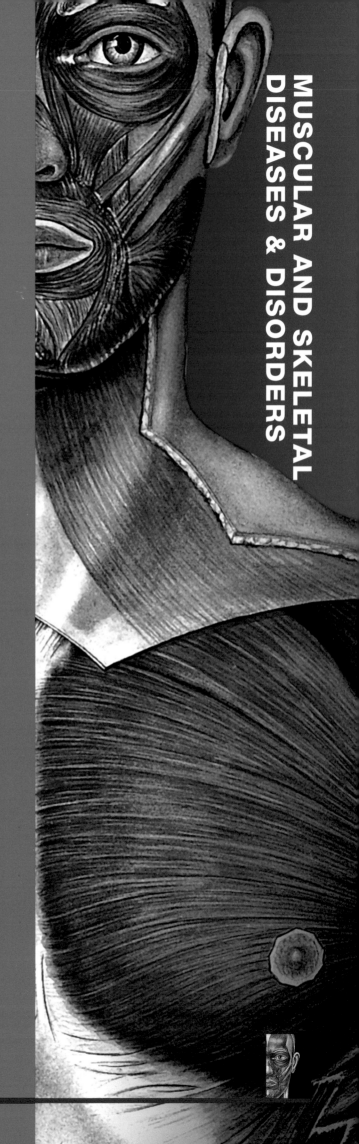

MUSCULAR AND SKELETAL DISEASES & DISORDERS

Osteoarthritis (OA)

- Most common type of arthritis.
- Primarily affects cartilage, the tissue that cushions the ends of bones within the joints.
- May initially affect joints asymmetrically.
- Affects hands and weight bearing joints.
- Can cause joint pain and stiffness.
- Usually develops slowly over many years.

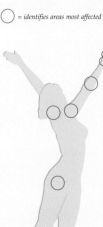

◯ = identifies areas most affected by OA.

Rheumatoid Arthritis (RA)

- Causes redness, warmth, and swelling of joints.
- Usually affects the same joint on both sides of the body.
- Often causes a general feeling of sickness, fatigue, weight loss, and fever.
- May develop suddenly, within weeks or months.
- Most often begins between ages 25 and 50.

◯ = identifies areas most affected by RA.

Other Arthritic Diseases

Many people use the word *arthritis* to refer to all rheumatic diseases. However, the word literally means joint inflammation. Other types of arthritis include:

Fibromyalgia (Fibrositis)

- Chronic disorder that causes pain throughout the tissues that support and move the bones and joints.
- Pain, stiffness, and localized tender points occur in the muscles and tendons, particularly those of the spine, shoulders, and hips.
- Patients may also experience fatigue and sleep disturbances.

Gout

- Results from deposits of needle-like crystals of uric acid in the joints.
- The crystals cause inflammation, swelling, and pain in the affected joint, which is often the big toe.

Juvenile Rheumatoid Arthritis

- Most common form of arthritis in children.
- Causes pain, stiffness, swelling, and impaired function of the joints.
- May be associated with rashes or fevers; may affect various parts of the body.

Systemic Lupus Erythematosus

- Also known as *lupus* or *SLE*.
- Can result in inflammation of and damage to the joints, skin, kidneys, heart, lungs, blood vessels, and brain.

Bursitis

- Inflammation of a bursa, a small, fluid-filled sac that absorbs shock and reduces friction around a joint.
- May be caused by arthritis in the joint or by injury or infection of the bursa.
- Produces pain and tenderness and may limit the movement of nearby joints.

Tendinitis

- Inflammation of a tendon, a cord of fibrous tissue that attaches muscle to bone.
- May be caused by overuse, injury, or a rheumatic condition.
- Produces pain and tenderness and may restrict movement of nearby joints.

Common Symptoms of Arthritis

- Swelling in one or more joints.
- Stiffness around the joints (each episode of stiffness for RA lasts one hour or more, but OA lasts 30 minutes or less).
- Constant or recurring pain or tenderness in a joint.
- Difficulty using or moving a joint normally.
- Warmth and redness in a joint.

If you have any of these symptoms for more than two weeks, contact your physician.

©2008 Wolters Kluwer Health | Lippincott Williams & Wilkins
Published by **Anatomical Chart Company, Skokie, IL**

Joints Affected by Osteoarthritis (OA)

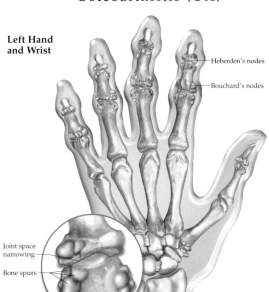

Left Hand and Wrist

- Heberden's nodes
- Bouchard's nodes
- Joint space narrowing
- Bone spurs

Joints Affected by Rheumatoid Arthritis (RA)

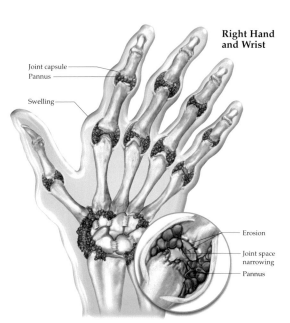

Right Hand and Wrist

- Joint capsule
- Pannus
- Swelling
- Erosion
- Joint space narrowing
- Pannus

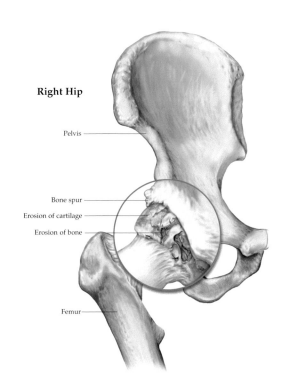

Right Hip

- Pelvis
- Bone spur
- Erosion of cartilage
- Erosion of bone
- Femur

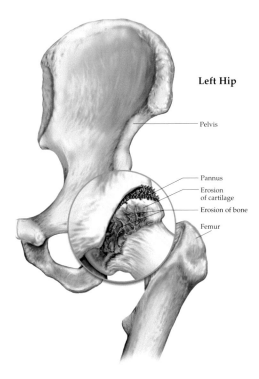

Left Hip

- Pelvis
- Pannus
- Erosion of cartilage
- Erosion of bone
- Femur

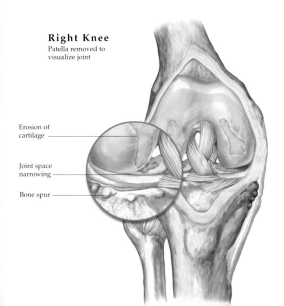

Right Knee
Patella removed to visualize joint

- Erosion of cartilage
- Joint space narrowing
- Bone spur

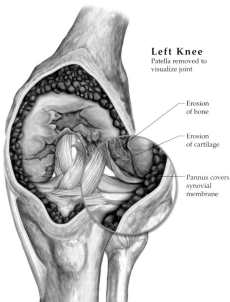

Left Knee
Patella removed to visualize joint

- Erosion of bone
- Erosion of cartilage
- Pannus covers synovial membrane

Understanding Carpal Tunnel Syndrome

52

Nerve Compression Syndromes

Continuous or periodic compression on a nerve can cause damage over time. Certain nerves are located in regions of the body that are especially vulnerable to compression injuries. The most common nerve compression disorder is Carpal Tunnel Syndrome.

Median nerve

Branches of median nerve

Flexor tendons

Carpal tunnel

Normal median nerve

What Is Carpal Tunnel Syndrome?

Carpal Tunnel Syndrome (CTS) is the pain, numbness and weakness associated with compression of the median nerve against the inelastic transverse carpal ligament. Often, this is caused by pressure from swollen synovium of the flexor tendons. If left untreated, CTS can lead to considerable discomfort, impaired function of the hand(s), and permanent disability. It is the most common hand disorder, affecting 1-5% of the general population.

The Carpal Tunnel

The carpal tunnel is a narrow, rigid passage formed by the carpal bones of the wrist and the tough, inelastic transverse carpal ligament. Traveling through the tunnel are nine flexor tendons and the median nerve. The flexor muscles originate in the forearm and attach, as tendons, to bones of the fingers and thumb. As these muscles contract to bend the fingers, the tendons slide through the carpal tunnel. The median nerve travels through the carpal tunnel and then divides into a motor branch that controls the thumb muscles, and sensory branches that provide over half of the hand with its sense of touch.

Cross Section of Normal Wrist

Carpal bones:
1. Trapezium
2. Trapezoid
3. Capitate
4. Hamate

Carpal tunnel

Cross Section of Wrist with CTS

Flexor tendons

Swollen synovium of tendons

Compressed median nerve

Transverse carpal ligament

Increased pressure on the median nerve decreases blood flow. The resulting lack of nutrients and oxygen causes disturbances in nerve conduction and early symptoms of CTS. If compression persists, the nerve begins to swell. The myelin sheath, which plays an important role in nerve conduction, begins to thin and degenerate.

Flexor tendon in synovium

Nerve fiber

Capillary plexus

Basal lamina

Degenerated myelin sheath

Axon of nerve

Normal myelin sheath

Synovium

Median nerve

Flexor muscles

Transverse carpal ligament

Ulnar nerve

Hook of hamate

Flexor tendons

Branches of median nerve

What Causes CTS?

CTS can be brought on by any factor contributing to increased pressure within the carpal tunnel. Often, several factors are present.

Systemic disorders: diabetes, rheumatoid arthritis, hypothyroidism, amyloidosis.

Repetitive trauma: repetitive movements expose the nerve to compression forces and stretching.

Erosion of bone and cartilage

Inflamed, swollen synovium

Compressed median nerve

Rheumatoid Arthritis

Flexor tendons

Median nerve

Repetitive Trauma

Tenosynovitis: thickening of the tendon synovium caused by mechanical stress put on sliding tendons during repetitive movements.

Transverse carpal ligament

Tendon

Swollen synovium

Other Causes:
Edema: increased fluid within the carpal tunnel due to tissue injury, congestive heart failure, or pregnancy.
Fractures, dislocations of the wrist: displaced bones or spurs disrupt the carpal tunnel.
Carpal tunnel size: inherited small bone structure may lead to increased incidence of CTS.

Healthy Lifestyle Changes

Avoid repetitive movements of the hands that are forceful, awkward, or involve pinching, grasping or extreme flexion or extension. If repetition is unavoidable, keep the wrist straight or slightly extended when hands are in motion. Maintain good posture, keep hands and arms warm, and take sufficient time to rest throughout the day. Never continue an activity that causes pain. Avoid high salt intake, which causes water retention, and smoking, which reduces blood flow.

Flexion
Nerve is compressed between tendons and transverse carpal ligament.

Neutral
Fluid, tendons, and nerve flow freely through tunnel.

Extension
Nerve is stretched over tendons and bones.

Symptoms
Paresthesia:
numbness and tingling ("pins and needles") in the hand.
Night pain:
relieved by shaking or exercising the hand. May occur several times a night.
Daytime pain:
aggravated by activity, more persistent as CTS progresses. May radiate up to forearm, elbow, or shoulder.
Thumb muscle weakness:
grasping and pinching are difficult. Hand feels stiff and clumsy. In severe cases, thumb muscles diminish in size.

Managing CTS
CTS is most manageable when diagnosed early, as its effects can lead to irreversible nerve damage over time. The goal of managing CTS is to decrease pressure on the median nerve.

Nonoperative measures:
reduce edema and inflammation of tissues
 • rest the hand(s)
 • wear a wrist splint
 • anti-inflammatory medications and diuretics
 • modify hand activity and work environment
 • steroid injections
 • treat underlying systemic diseases

In more severe cases of CTS it may be necessary to diminish pressure on the nerve and increase the size of the carpal tunnel by surgically dividing the transverse carpal ligament.

Crucial to the healing process and sustained relief is a highly motivated patient willing to modify his or her lifestyle or work environment to eliminate repeated stress on the hands.

Risk Factors
Female
40 or older
Job or hobbies involve highly repetitive tasks
Diabetes
Rheumatoid arthritis
Hypothyroidism
Pregnancy
Trauma to wrist
Menopause
Obesity

Anatomy and Injuries of the Foot and Ankle

53

NORMAL ANATOMY

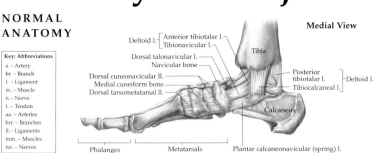

Medial View

Deltoid l.
Anterior tibiotalar l.
Tibionavicular l.
Dorsal talonavicular l.
Navicular bone
Dorsal cuneonavicular ll.
Medial cuneiform bone
Dorsal tarsometatarsal ll.
Tibia
Posterior tibiotalar l.
Tibiocalcaneal l.
Deltoid l.
Calcaneus
Phalanges
Metatarsals
Plantar calcaneonavicular (spring) l.

Key: Abbreviations
a. – Artery
br. – Branch
l. – Ligament
m. – Muscle
n. – Nerve
t. – Tendon
aa. – Arteries
brr. – Branches
ll. – Ligaments
mm. – Muscles
nn. – Nerves

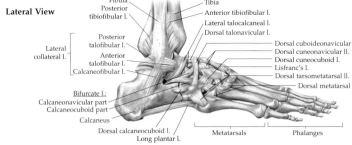

Lateral View

Fibula
Posterior tibiofibular l.
Tibia
Anterior tibiofibular l.
Lateral talocalcaneal l.
Dorsal talonavicular l.
Posterior talofibular l.
Lateral collateral l.
Anterior talofibular l.
Calcaneofibular l.
Dorsal cuboideonavicular l.
Dorsal cuneonavicular ll.
Dorsal cuneocuboid l.
Lisfranc's l.
Dorsal tarsometatarsal ll.
Dorsal metatarsal ll.
Bifurcate l.:
Calcaneonavicular part
Calcaneocuboid part
Calcaneus
Dorsal calcaneocuboid l.
Long plantar l.
Metatarsals
Phalanges

NERVE AND BLOOD SUPPLY

Key: Arteries and Nerves

1. Superficial peroneal n.
2. Deep peroneal n.
3. Intermediate dorsal cutaneous n.
4. Medial dorsal cutaneous n.
5. Anterior tibial a.
6. Perforating br. of peroneal a.
7. Lateral malleolar a.
8. Lateral malleolar network
9. Lateral calcaneal brr. of sural n.
10. Lateral br. of deep peroneal n.
11. Lateral tarsal a.
12. Arcuate a.
13. Lateral dorsal cutaneous br. of sural n.
14. Dorsal digital brr. of superficial peroneal n.
15. Dorsal digital brr. of deep peroneal n.
16. Dorsal digital aa.
17. Anterior perforating aa.
18. Deep plantar a.
19. Posterior perforating aa.
20. Medial br. of deep peroneal n.
21. Medial tarsal aa.
22. Dorsalis pedis a.
23. Posterior tibial a. & n.
24. Calcaneal br. of posterior tibial a.
25. Medial malleolar a.
26. Lateral plantar a. & n.
27. Medial plantar a. & n.
28. Medial calcaneal brr. of sural n.
29. Deep plantar arch
30. Superficial br. of lateral plantar n.
31. Plantar metatarsal aa.
32. Common plantar digital nn.
33. Plantar digital brr. of lateral plantar n.
34. Plantar digital brr. of medial plantar n.
35. Proper plantar digital aa.
36. Superficial brr. of medial plantar a. & n.

Plantar View

Calcaneus
Spring ll.
Tibialis posterior t.
Tibialis anterior t.
Long plantar l.
Peroneus longus t.
Peroneus brevis t.

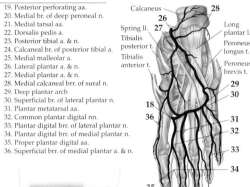
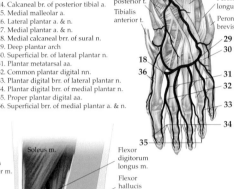

Soleus m.
Extensor digitorum longus m.
Tibialis anterior m.
Soleus m.
Flexor digitorum longus m.
Flexor hallucis longus m.
Tibia
Achilles t.
Tarsal tunnel
Tibialis posterior t.
Tibialis anterior t.
Flexor digitorum longus t.
Flexor hallucis longus t.
Peroneus longus m.
Fibula
Peroneus brevis t.
Retinaculum
Peroneus tertius t.
Extensor hallucis longus t.

FOOT INJURIES

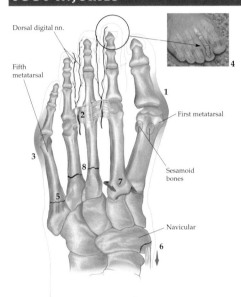

Dorsal digital nn.
Fifth metatarsal
First metatarsal
Sesamoid bones
Navicular

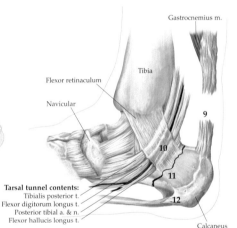

Gastrocnemius m.
Flexor retinaculum
Navicular
Tibia
Tarsal tunnel contents:
Tibialis posterior t.
Flexor digitorum longus t.
Posterior tibial a. & n.
Flexor hallucis longus t.
Calcaneus

Forefoot Injuries

1. **BUNION** – The misalignment of the bones of the big toe (*first metatarsal and sesamoid bones*) is often caused by ill-fitting shoes. Symptoms include a bulge on the inside of the foot with pain, redness, and swelling.
2. **MORTON'S NEUROMA** – A neuroma is a noncancerous thickening of nerve tissue; this type occurs in a nerve between the third and fourth toes. It causes sharp and burning pain in the ball of the foot and toes and sometimes numbness. It is often caused by ill-fitting shoes.
3. **BUNIONETTE** (*Tailor's bunion*) – Similar to a bunion, but this involves the little toe.
4. **HAMMERTOE** – A permanent sideways bend in a middle toe joint. Aggravation by tight shoes results in pain over the prominent bony areas of the toe. A hard corn may develop over this prominence as well.

Midfoot Injuries

5. **JONES' FRACTURE** – A fracture of the base of the little toe (*fifth metatarsal bone*). People often experience pain and swelling over the middle/outside area of the midportion of the foot.
6. **CHOPART AVULSION FRACTURE** – An ankle-twisting injury that may tear the tendon attached to the navicular bone and pull a small piece of the bone away.
7. **LISFRANC DISLOCATION** – This is a relatively rare condition that is often misdiagnosed. A twisting fall can dislodge the second bone from the first because the first and second metatarsal bones are not held together well.
8. **METATARSAL STRESS FRACTURE** – A common cause of foot pain when people suddenly increase their activities (*e.g. taking up jogging*). Excessive stress on all of the foot can cause this hairline break resulting in pain and swelling.

Hindfoot Injuries

9. **ACHILLES' TENDON RUPTURE** – Often a sports-related injury for those who suddenly take up activity or are active only on the weekends. A "pop" is often felt in the posterior ankle, with edema (swelling) and pain.
10. **TARSAL TUNNEL SYNDROME** – Most commonly, the entrapment of the tibial nerve by the flexor retinaculum. Pain and stiffness occur over this area on the inside part of the ankle.
11. **CALCANEAL FRACTURE** – A break in the "heel bone" commonly caused by a high fall (e.g. it is becoming more common amongst snowboarders).
12. **PLANTAR FASCIITIS WITH HEEL SPURS** – The most common cause of heel pain is inflammation of the connective tissue on the sole of the foot (plantar fascia). It is often associated with a bony protrusion known as a heel spur.

SPRAINS AND FRACTURES

Common Sprain Sites

Anterior talofibular l.
Calcaneofibular l.
Deltoid l.

Common Fracture Sites

Key:
A – Tibial plafond
B – Malleolar
C – Osteochondral fracture of the talar dome
D – Jones' fracture
E – Metatarsal stress fracture
F – Maisonneuve

A
B
B
C
D
E
F

* There are two sites of fracture in this type.

IMPINGEMENT

Anterior Impingement Syndrome

Impingement injuries often occur secondarily to traumatic injuries (such as sprains), infections, or degenerative disease states. A tendency toward this type of malady is also inherited.

Normal Anatomy
(Neutral position)

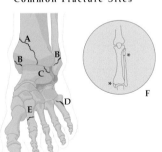

Talocrural joint
Tibia
Talus
Calcaneus

Dorsiflexed Ankle Causing Impingement

Repeated impact between the anterior tibia and dorsal tarsal bone can cause the formation of osteophytes, or bone spurs. This is a painful condition that causes joint stiffness and immobility.

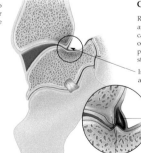

Impingement of synovial fluid and joint capsule
Inflamed synovium
Bone spurs

MOVEMENT ABOUT THE ANKLE

Inversion
An inward rotation of the ankle joint. Severe or sudden inversion can cause sprains of ligaments and fractures of the foot bones. *For example:* Jones' fracture, Chopart avulsion fracture, tears of the anterior talofibular or calcaneofibular ligament.

Eversion
An outward rotation of the ankle joint. Severe or sudden eversion can cause sprains of the foot ligaments. *For example:* Deltoid ligament tears.

Dorsiflexion
Upward flexion of the ankle joint. Constant repetition of this movement can cause injury. *For example:* Soccer players may develop dorsal ankle impingement (*see above*) from repetitive kicking motions.

Plantar Flexion
Downward flexion of the ankle joint. Constant repetition of this movement can cause injury. *For example:* Ballet dancers can acquire posterior ankle impingement syndrome (*see above*) from being "on point" too often.

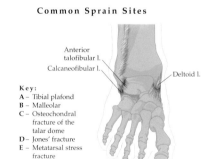
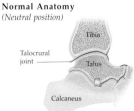

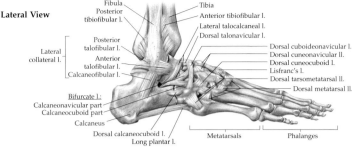

©2008 Wolters Kluwer Health | Lippincott Williams & Wilkins | Published by Anatomical Chart Company, Skokie, IL

Anatomy and Injuries of the Hand & Wrist

54

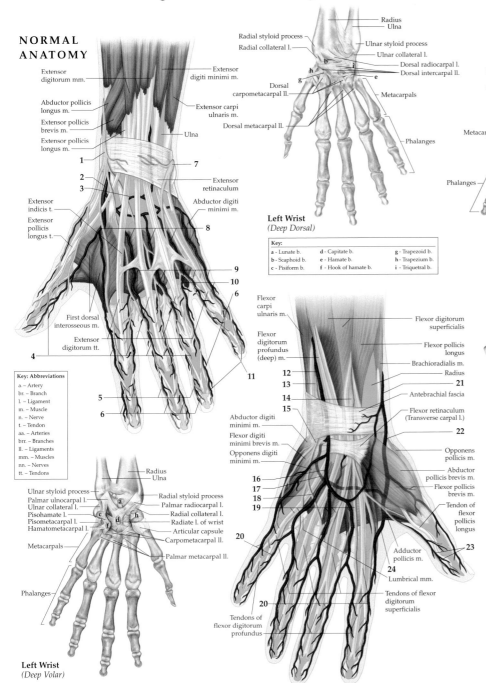

NORMAL ANATOMY

Extensor digitorum mm.
Abductor pollicis longus m.
Extensor pollicis brevis m.
Extensor pollicis longus m.
Extensor indicis t.
Extensor pollicis longus t.
First dorsal interosseous m.
Extensor digitorum tt.
Extensor digiti minimi m.
Extensor carpi ulnaris m.
Ulna
Extensor retinaculum
Abductor digiti minimi m.

1
7
2
3
8
9
10
6
4
5
6
11

Radius
Ulna
Radial styloid process
Radial collateral l.
Dorsal carpometacarpal ll.
Dorsal metacarpal ll.
Ulnar styloid process
Ulnar collateral l.
Dorsal radiocarpal l.
Dorsal intercarpal ll.
Metacarpals
Phalanges

Left Wrist
(Deep Dorsal)

Key:
a – Lunate b. d – Capitate b. g – Trapezoid b.
b – Scaphoid b. e – Hamate b. h – Trapezium b.
c – Pisiform b. f – Hook of hamate b. i – Triquetral b.

Key: Abbreviations
a. – Artery
br. – Branch
l. – Ligament
m. – Muscle
n. – Nerve
t. – Tendon
aa. – Arteries
brr. – Branches
ll. – Ligaments
mm. – Muscles
nn. – Nerves
tt. – Tendons

Radius
Ulna
Ulnar styloid process
Palmar ulnocarpal l.
Ulnar collateral l.
Pisohamate l.
Pisometacarpal l.
Hamatometacarpal l.
Metacarpals
Phalanges
Radial styloid process
Palmar radiocarpal l.
Radial collateral l.
Radiate l. of wrist
Articular capsule
Carpometacarpal ll.
Palmar metacarpal ll.

Left Wrist
(Deep Volar)

Flexor carpi ulnaris m.
Flexor digitorum profundus (deep) m.
Abductor digiti minimi m.
Flexor digiti minimi brevis m.
Opponens digiti minimi m.
Flexor digitorum superficialis
Flexor pollicis longus
Brachioradialis m.
Radius
Antebrachial fascia
Flexor retinaculum (Transverse carpal l.)
Opponens pollicis m.
Abductor pollicis brevis m.
Flexor pollicis brevis m.
Tendon of flexor pollicis longus
Adductor pollicis m.
Lumbrical mm.
Tendons of flexor digitorum superficialis
Tendons of flexor digitorum profundus

12 13 14 15 16 17 18 19 20 21 22 23 24 20

Key: Arteries and Nerves
1. Radial n., superficial br.
2. Radial a.
3. Dorsal carpal arterial arch
4. Dorsal digital brr., radial n.
5. Median n., dorsal brr. of proper digital nn.
6. Dorsal brr. of proper palmar digital aa.
7. Ulnar n., dorsal br.
8. Dorsal metacarpal aa.
9. Digital aa.
10. Dorsal digital brr., ulnar n.
11. Dorsal brr. of proper palmar digital nn.
12. Ulnar a.
13. Ulnar n.
14. Median n.
15. Ulnar n., superficial br.
16. Superficial palmar arch
17. Deep palmar arch
18. Communicating br. of median n. with ulnar n.
19. Common palmar digital aa. & nn.
20. Proper palmar digital aa. & nn.
21. Radial a.
22. Radial a., superficial br.
23. Proper digital a. & n. to thumb
24. Radialis indicis a.

FRACTURES

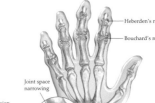

Left Hand *(Palmar/Volar)*
Radius
Lunate
Capitate
Metacarpals
Phalanges
Scaphoid *(60% of all wrist fractures)*

Hand Fractures

Radial styloid
Keypunch

Radial Fractures

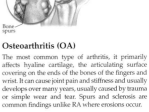

Scaphoid
Radius

Colles' fracture *(extra-articular dorsal angulation)*
Barton's fracture *(intra-articular dorsal fragment)*
Smith's fracture *(extra-articular volar angulation)*

Left Hand *(Lateral)*

HAND AND WRIST INJURIES

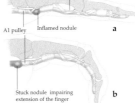

Joint capsule
Pannus
Swelling
Erosion
Joint space narrowing
Pannus

Heberden's nodes
Bouchard's nodes
Joint space narrowing
Bone spurs

Rheumatoid Arthritis (RA)
A chronic disease that develops over weeks or months, most often between the ages of 25 and 50, it causes a general feeling of sickness, plus fatigue, weight loss, and fever. This type of arthritis usually affects the same joint on both sides of the body with redness, warmth, and swelling. Deformity occurs in later stages of the disease.

Osteoarthritis (OA)
The most common type of arthritis, it primarily affects hyaline cartilage, the articulating surface covering on the ends of the bones of the fingers and wrist. It can cause joint pain and stiffness and usually develops over many years, usually caused by trauma or simple wear and tear. Spurs and sclerosis are common findings unlike RA where erosions occur.

Carpal Tunnel Syndrome (CTS)

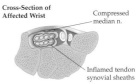

Normal Wrist Cross-Section
Median n.
Flexor retinaculum
Carpal bones
Flexor tendons

Cross-Section of Affected Wrist
Compressed median n.
Inflamed tendon synovial sheaths

This common disorder causes pain, numbness, and weakness in the hand and is associated with compression of the median nerve against the inelastic transverse carpal ligament in the wrist. Continuous or periodic compression on the nerve can cause damage over time. It has a variety of causes, but it is most commonly caused by repetitive movements (e.g., typing on a keyboard) that expose the nerve to compression forces and stretching.

Finger Maladies

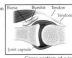

Tendon
A1 pulley
Inflamed nodule
a
Stuck nodule impairing extension of the finger
b

Bursitis - inflammation of a bursa; a sack that separates bone from muscle near a joint.
Tendonitis - inflammation of a tendon.
Bursa Bursitis Tendon
Joint capsule
Cross-section of a joint

Trigger Finger
A type of tenosynovitis (inflammation of the tendon and synovium), it is characterized by the inability to extend a finger after it has been flexed (b). An inflamed nodule in the tendon is trapped proximal to the first flexor tendon pulley.

Cyst that has ballooned out from a defect in the synovial membrane of the carpometacarpal joint
Third metacarpal
Capitate Synovial membrane

Ganglion Cyst
Occurring most often on the back of the wrist or hand, this sac is filled with the synovial fluid from a nearby joint. It is a hernia of the joint's capsule that causes the bulge. A volar wrist ganglion is less common.

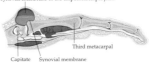

Extensor pollicis brevis t.
Scaphoid
Adductor pollicis
Extensor pollicis longus t.
Extensor retinaculum
Superficial brr. of radial n.
Radial a.
Bursitis
DeQuervain's tenosynovitis

Snuffbox Tenderness
The anatomical snuffbox is a superficial concavity near the radius (R) that is bound by tendons of the thumb. The radial artery passes through this space. The tendon sheaths that pass beneath the extensor retinaculum can become inflamed, causing tenderness and swelling, or DeQuervain's tenosynovitis. Another very common cause of pain in this region is a fracture of the scaphoid bone.

MOVEMENT ABOUT THE WRIST AND FINGERS

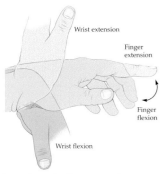

Wrist extension
Finger extension
Finger flexion
Wrist flexion

Flexion/Extension/Hyperextension
These movements occur between the forearm bones *(radius and ulna)* and the carpal bones of the wrist. The most common cause of wrist trauma is a fall on an extended wrist (e.g., Colles', Barton's, scaphoid fractures). Hyperextension of the fingers can lead to dislocation and ligament injuries on the volar aspect of the finger.

Supination/Pronation
Supination is the act of turning you palm face-up ("holds soup"), while pronation is turning your hand down facing the floor. Falls on an outstretched hand in extreme pronation have been associated with dorsal dislocations at the radio-ulnar (wrist) joint. A fall with the hand outstretched in a supinated position can cause a fracture of the radius (R) or volar dislocation of the radio-ulnar joint.

Supination Pronation

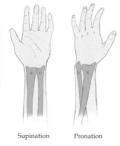

Thumb Opposition
The ability to touch the thumb to the fifth digit (pinky finger) is the human being's unique advantage in the animal kingdom. It allows us to perform many ordinary, but essential, daily tasks, such as holding a pen or eating with a fork. Any injury to the median nerve *(including carpal tunnel syndrome)* inhibits our ability to use the thumb in this manner.

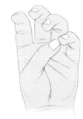

Anatomy and Injuries of the Hip

55

Normal Anatomy of the Hip Region

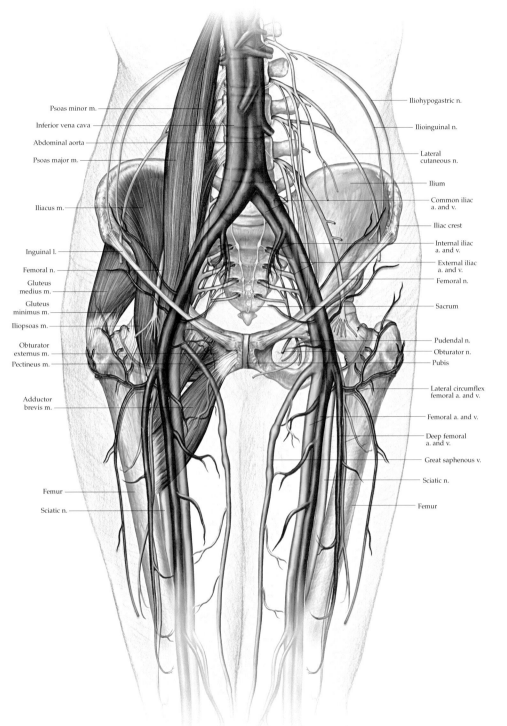

- Psoas minor m.
- Inferior vena cava
- Abdominal aorta
- Psoas major m.
- Iliacus m.
- Inguinal l.
- Femoral n.
- Gluteus medius m.
- Gluteus minimus m.
- Iliopsoas m.
- Obturator externus m.
- Pectineus m.
- Adductor brevis m.
- Femur
- Sciatic n.

- Iliohypogastric n.
- Ilioinguinal n.
- Lateral cutaneous n.
- Ilium
- Common iliac a. and v.
- Iliac crest
- Internal iliac a. and v.
- External iliac a. and v.
- Femoral n.
- Sacrum
- Pudendal n.
- Obturator n.
- Pubis
- Lateral circumflex femoral a. and v.
- Femoral a. and v.
- Deep femoral a. and v.
- Great saphenous v.
- Sciatic n.
- Femur

BLOOD SUPPLY AND INJURIES

Cross-section of Hip Joint Area

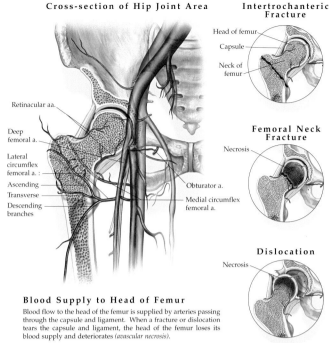

- Retinacular aa.
- Deep femoral a.
- Lateral circumflex femoral a. :
- Ascending
- Transverse
- Descending branches
- Obturator a.
- Medial circumflex femoral a.

Intertrochanteric Fracture
- Head of femur
- Capsule
- Neck of femur

Femoral Neck Fracture
- Necrosis

Dislocation
- Necrosis

Blood Supply to Head of Femur

Blood flow to the head of the femur is supplied by arteries passing through the capsule and ligament. When a fracture or dislocation tears the capsule and ligament, the head of the femur loses its blood supply and deteriorates (avascular necrosis).

HIP JOINT FRACTURES

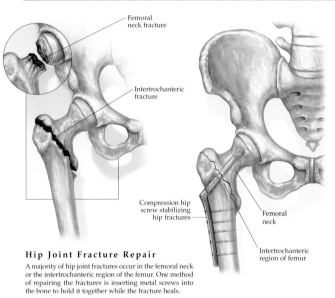

- Femoral neck fracture
- Intertrochanteric fracture
- Compression hip screw stabilizing hip fractures
- Femoral neck
- Intertrochanteric region of femur

Hip Joint Fracture Repair

A majority of hip joint fractures occur in the femoral neck or the intertrochanteric region of the femur. One method of repairing the fractures is inserting metal screws into the bone to hold it together while the fracture heals.

TOTAL HIP ARTHROPLASTY (REPLACEMENT)

Degenerative changes of the joint cartilage may lead to fragmentation, thinning or erosive changes. These arthritic changes can be treated with a total hip arthroplasty (replacement).

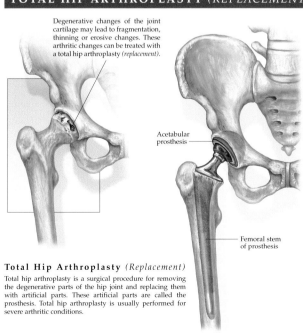

- Acetabular prosthesis
- Femoral stem of prosthesis

Total Hip Arthroplasty (Replacement)

Total hip arthroplasty is a surgical procedure for removing the degenerative parts of the hip joint and replacing them with artificial parts. These artificial parts are called the prosthesis. Total hip arthroplasty is usually performed for severe arthritic conditions.

Anterior View of Hip Joint
Posterior View of Hip Joint
Lateral View of Hip Joint (Opened)

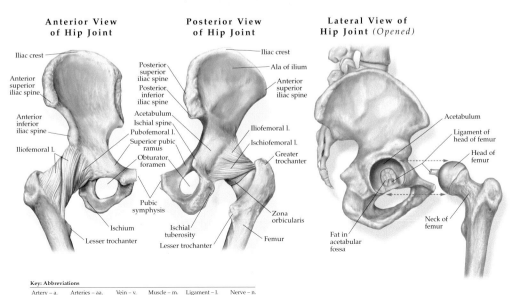

- Iliac crest
- Anterior superior iliac spine
- Anterior inferior iliac spine
- Iliofemoral l.
- Ischium
- Lesser trochanter

- Posterior superior iliac spine
- Posterior inferior iliac spine
- Acetabulum
- Ischial spine
- Pubofemoral l.
- Superior pubic ramus
- Obturator foramen
- Pubic symphysis
- Ischial tuberosity
- Lesser trochanter

- Iliac crest
- Ala of ilium
- Anterior superior iliac spine
- Iliofemoral l.
- Ischiofemoral l.
- Greater trochanter
- Zona orbicularis
- Femur

- Acetabulum
- Ligament of head of femur
- Head of femur
- Neck of femur
- Fat in acetabular fossa

Key: Abbreviations

Artery – a.   Arteries – aa.   Vein – v.   Muscle – m.   Ligament – l.   Nerve – n.

Hip and Knee Inflammations

56

Normal Anatomy

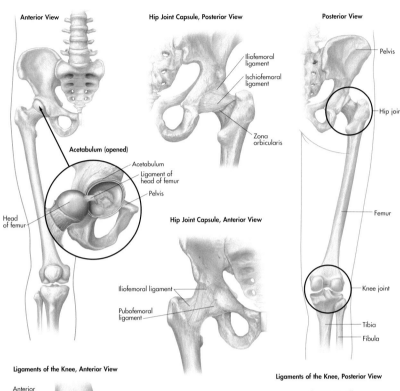

Anterior View

Hip Joint Capsule, Posterior View
- Iliofemoral ligament
- Ischiofemoral ligament
- Zona orbicularis

Posterior View
- Pelvis
- Hip joint
- Femur
- Knee joint
- Tibia
- Fibula

Acetabulum (opened)
- Acetabulum
- Ligament of head of femur
- Pelvis
- Head of femur

Hip Joint Capsule, Anterior View
- Iliofemoral ligament
- Pubofemoral ligament

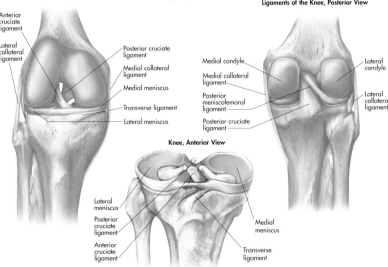

Ligaments of the Knee, Anterior View
- Anterior cruciate ligament
- Lateral collateral ligament
- Posterior cruciate ligament
- Medial collateral ligament
- Medial meniscus
- Transverse ligament
- Lateral meniscus

Ligaments of the Knee, Posterior View
- Medial condyle
- Medial collateral ligament
- Posterior meniscofemoral ligament
- Posterior cruciate ligament
- Lateral condyle
- Lateral collateral ligament

Knee, Anterior View
- Lateral meniscus
- Posterior cruciate ligament
- Anterior cruciate ligament
- Medial meniscus
- Transverse ligament

Bursitis

A bursa is a fluid-filled sac that helps to cushion and lubricate body's joints (tendons, ligaments, muscles, and bones). Bursitis is a painful swelling of a bursa. People who repeatedly overuse or stress the same areas around the joints, whether it is related to their jobs, sports, or daily activities, have a greater chance of developing bursitis.

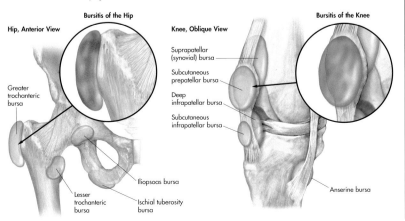

Bursitis of the Hip

Hip, Anterior View
- Greater trochanteric bursa
- Lesser trochanteric bursa
- Iliopsoas bursa
- Ischial tuberosity bursa

Knee, Oblique View
- Suprapatellar (synovial) bursa
- Subcutaneous prepatellar bursa
- Deep infrapatellar bursa
- Subcutaneous infrapatellar bursa
- Anserine bursa

Bursitis of the Knee

Osteoarthritis (OA)

Osteoarthritis is the most common type of arthritis (inflammation of a joint). It can lead to degenerative joint disease and significant disability. OA is associated with breakdown of the hyaline cartilage, which protects the surface of the joints during movement. It occurs most commonly in the weight bearing joints of the hips and knees, but it is also a common cause of chronic lower back or spine pain. OA usually does not affect other joints, unless prior injury or excessive stress is involved. OA is essentially caused by a lifetime of wear and tear of the joints involved, but genetics may also play a role.

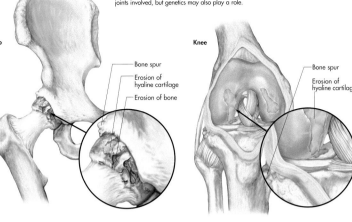

Hip
- Bone spur
- Erosion of hyaline cartilage
- Erosion of bone

Knee
- Bone spur
- Erosion of hyaline cartilage

Rheumatoid Arthritis (RA)

Rheumatoid arthritis is a chronic disease of the joints that causes diffuse joint degeneration. RA causes inflammation of the synovium (tissue lining the joints), which can eventually lead to the destruction of the hyaline cartilage of the joints. Joints of the hands, wrists, elbows, feet, ankles, knees, or neck are usually affected. However, in extreme cases, RA may also affect other parts of the body (heart, lungs, nerves, eyes, or blood vessels). The cause of rheumatoid arthritis is unknown, but it is an autoimmune disease.

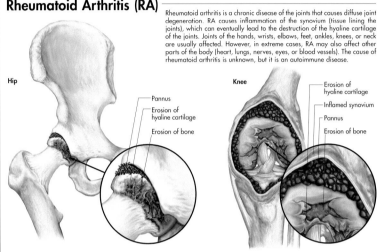

Hip
- Pannus
- Erosion of hyaline cartilage
- Erosion of bone

Knee
- Erosion of hyaline cartilage
- Inflamed synovium
- Pannus
- Erosion of bone

Gout and Pseudogout

Gout and pseudogout are other forms of joint inflammation. These are the body's reaction to the presence of irritating crystal deposits, uric acid (gout) and calcium pyrophospate (pseudogout), in the joints. The pain can be intense, but treatment is usually effective in alleviating this pain. Mild cases may be controlled by diet alone. However, recurring attacks of gout or pseudogout may require long-term medication to prevent damage to bones, cartilages, and the kidneys.

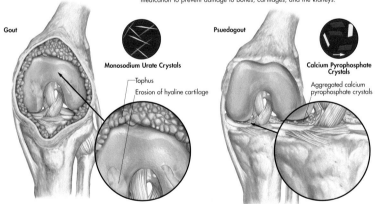

Gout
- Monosodium Urate Crystals
- Tophus
- Erosion of hyaline cartilage

Psuedogout
- Calcium Pyrophosphate Crystals
- Aggregated calcium pyrophosphate crystals

Tendinopathy

Tendinopathy represents pathologic changes of the tendon; it is usually related to its chronic overuse. Since actual inflammation is rarely present, the use of the term "tendinitis" in defining tendinopathy has been discarded. Tendinopathy is characterized by microtears, degeneration of the collagen fibers with replacement of scar tissues (known as angiofibroblastic dysplasia), and apoptosis of the tenocytes (premature death of the tendon cells). Tendinopathy commonly occurs at the patellar tendon (jumper's knee), Achilles' tendon, lateral epicondyle (tennis elbow), and rotator cuff.

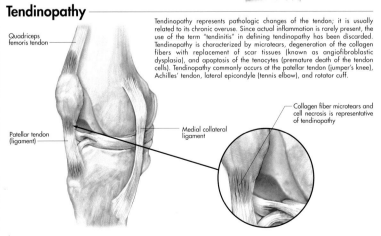

- Quadriceps femoris tendon
- Patellar tendon (ligament)
- Medial collateral ligament
- Collagen fiber microtears and cell necrosis is representative of tendinopathy

©2008 Wolters Kluwer | Lippincott Williams & Wilkins | Published by Anatomical Chart Company, Skokie, IL

Knee Injuries

57

Anterior View of Normal Knee
(Patella removed)

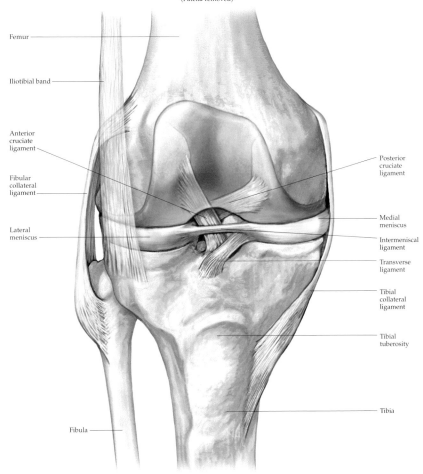

- Femur
- Iliotibial band
- Anterior cruciate ligament
- Fibular collateral ligament
- Lateral meniscus
- Fibula
- Posterior cruciate ligament
- Medial meniscus
- Intermeniscal ligament
- Transverse ligament
- Tibial collateral ligament
- Tibial tuberosity
- Tibia

Oblique View

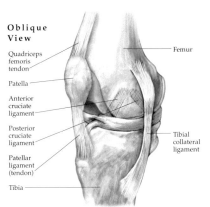

- Femur
- Quadriceps femoris tendon
- Patella
- Anterior cruciate ligament
- Posterior cruciate ligament
- Patellar ligament (tendon)
- Tibia
- Tibial collateral ligament

Posterior View

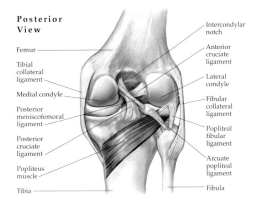

- Femur
- Tibial collateral ligament
- Medial condyle
- Posterior meniscofemoral ligament
- Posterior cruciate ligament
- Popliteus muscle
- Tibia
- Intercondylar notch
- Anterior cruciate ligament
- Lateral condyle
- Fibular collateral ligament
- Popliteal fibular ligament
- Arcuate popliteal ligament
- Fibula

Traumatic Knee Injuries

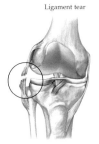 Ligament tear

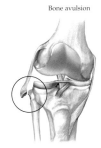 Bone avulsion

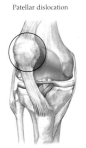 Ligament sprain

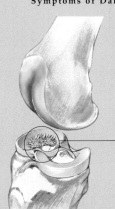 Patellar dislocation

Sports Related Ligament Injuries

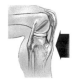

Sudden posterior movement of the tibia while the knee is flexed at 90 degree may damage the posterior cruciate ligament.

Hyperextension of the knee joint can damage the anterior cruciate and tibial collateral ligaments.

Forcible external rotation of the foot in the "whip-kick" causes the lower leg to twist at the knee, putting excessive strain on the tibial collateral ligament. It can also cause plical irritation or exacerbate patellar instability.

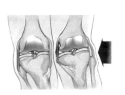

A lateral blow to the knees while the feet are firmly planted may cause damage to the tibial and fibular collateral ligaments.

Meniscus

The meniscus is a crescent-shaped piece of cartilage that lies between the femur and tibia. Each knee has two menisci, one medial and one lateral. Together, they cushion the joint by distributing downward forces outward and away from the central anchor points of the menisci.

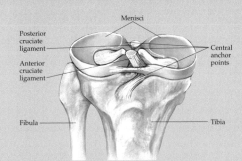

- Posterior cruciate ligament
- Anterior cruciate ligament
- Fibula
- Menisci
- Central anchor points
- Tibia

Meniscus Tears

Rotation of the femur can pinch and tear the meniscus.

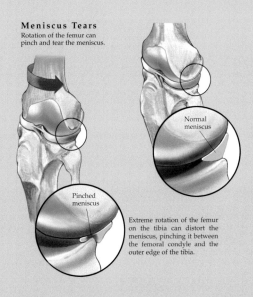

- Normal meniscus
- Pinched meniscus

Extreme rotation of the femur on the tibia can distort the meniscus, pinching it between the femoral condyle and the outer edge of the tibia.

Types of Meniscus Tears

Oblique | Longitudinal | Radial | Degenerative fraying

Symptoms of Damaged Menisci

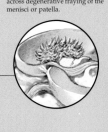

With your hand on your knee, you may feel roughness during a range of motion. This commonly occurs when the femur is gliding across degenerative fraying of the menisci or patella.

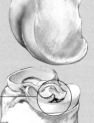
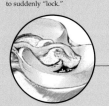
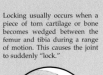

Locking usually occurs when a piece of torn cartilage or bone becomes wedged between the femur and tibia during a range of motion. This causes the joint to suddenly "lock."

Normal Anatomy of the Shoulder Anterior View

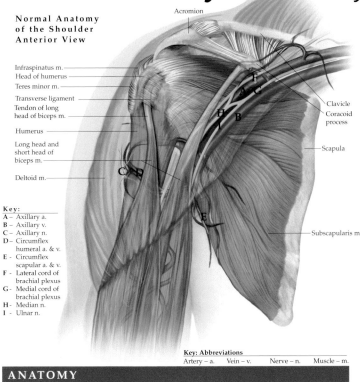

Infraspinatus m.
Head of humerus
Teres minor m.
Transverse ligament
Tendon of long head of biceps m.
Humerus
Long head and short head of biceps m.
Deltoid m.
Acromion
Clavicle
Coracoid process
Scapula
Subscapularis m.

Key:
A – Axillary a.
B – Axillary v.
C – Axillary n.
D – Circumflex humeral a. & v.
E - Circumflex scapular a. & v.
F - Lateral cord of brachial plexus
G - Medial cord of brachial plexus
H - Median n.
I - Ulnar n.

Key: Abbreviations
Artery – a.   Vein – v.   Nerve – n.   Muscle – m.

ANATOMY

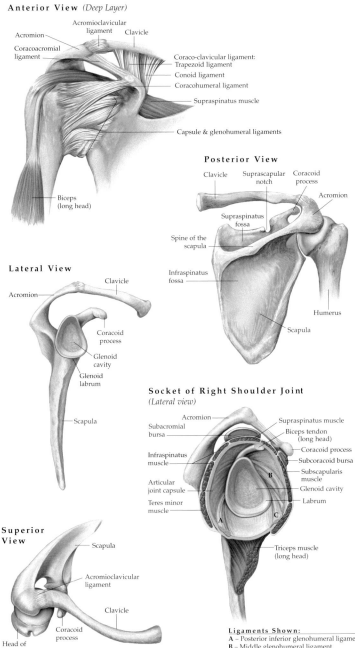

Anterior View (Deep Layer)

Acromion
Coracoacromial ligament
Acromioclavicular ligament
Clavicle
Coraco-clavicular ligament:
Trapezoid ligament
Conoid ligament
Coracohumeral ligament
Supraspinatus muscle
Capsule & glenohumeral ligaments
Biceps (long head)

Posterior View

Clavicle
Suprascapular notch
Coracoid process
Acromion
Supraspinatus fossa
Spine of the scapula
Infraspinatus fossa
Humerus
Scapula

Lateral View

Clavicle
Acromion
Coracoid process
Glenoid cavity
Glenoid labrum
Scapula

Socket of Right Shoulder Joint
(Lateral view)

Acromion
Subacromial bursa
Infraspinatus muscle
Articular joint capsule
Teres minor muscle
Supraspinatus muscle
Biceps tendon (long head)
Coracoid process
Subcoracoid bursa
Subscapularis muscle
Glenoid cavity
Labrum
Triceps muscle (long head)

Ligaments Shown:
A – Posterior inferior glenohumeral ligament
B – Middle glenohumeral ligament
C – Anterior inferior glenohumeral ligament

Superior View

Scapula
Acromioclavicular ligament
Clavicle
Coracoid process
Head of humerus

IMPINGEMENT

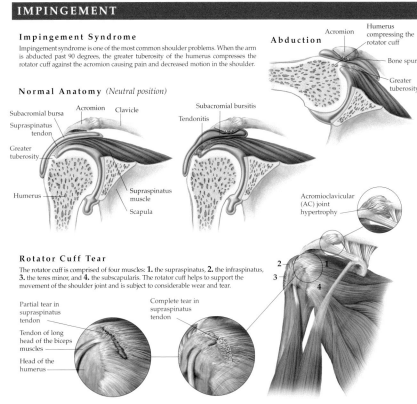

Impingement Syndrome
Impingement syndrome is one of the most common shoulder problems. When the arm is abducted past 90 degrees, the greater tuberosity of the humerus compresses the rotator cuff against the acromion causing pain and decreased motion in the shoulder.

Normal Anatomy (Neutral position)

Subacromial bursa
Acromion
Clavicle
Supraspinatus tendon
Greater tuberosity
Humerus
Supraspinatus muscle
Scapula
Subacromial bursitis
Tendonitis

Abduction
Acromion
Humerus compressing the rotator cuff
Bone spurs
Greater tuberosity

Acromioclavicular (AC) joint hypertrophy

Rotator Cuff Tear
The rotator cuff is comprised of four muscles: **1.** the supraspinatus, **2.** the infraspinatus, **3.** the teres minor, and **4.** the subscapularis. The rotator cuff helps to support the movement of the shoulder joint and is subject to considerable wear and tear.

Partial tear in supraspinatus tendon
Complete tear in supraspinatus tendon
Tendon of long head of the biceps muscles
Head of the humerus

TRAUMA

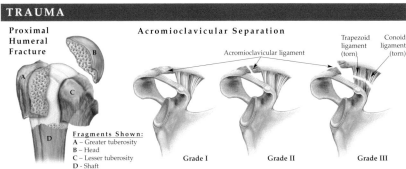

Proximal Humeral Fracture

Fragments Shown:
A – Greater tuberosity
B – Head
C – Lesser tuberosity
D - Shaft

Acromioclavicular Separation

Acromioclavicular ligament
Trapezoid ligament (torn)
Conoid ligament (torn)

Grade I   Grade II   Grade III

BICIPITAL TENDON PROBLEMS

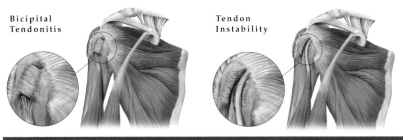

Bicipital Tendonitis

Tendon Instability

INSTABILITY

Bankart Lesion

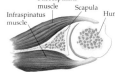

Labrum
Tear in Labrum

Dislocation of the Humerus
The shoulder joint is the most frequently dislocated joint in the body. It can become dislocated when a strong force pulls the shoulder outward (abduction) or when extreme rotation of the joint causes the head of the humerus to pop out of the shoulder socket.

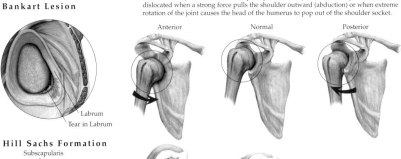

Anterior   Normal   Posterior

Hill Sachs Formation

Subscapularis muscle
Infraspinatus muscle
Scapula
Humerus

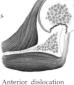

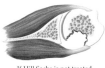

Normal shoulder anatomy viewed from above.

Anterior dislocation causes a piece of the humerus to break off.

Frequent dislocations cause the damaged area to enlarge.

If Hill Sachs is not treated, it can lead to chronic dislocations.

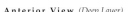

Human Spine Disorders

59

Anatomy

A Typical Cervical Vertebra (Superior View)

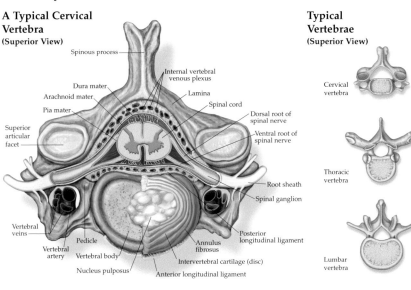

Spinous process
Internal vertebral venous plexus
Dura mater
Arachnoid mater
Pia mater
Lamina
Spinal cord
Dorsal root of spinal nerve
Ventral root of spinal nerve
Superior articular facet
Root sheath
Spinal ganglion
Vertebral veins
Pedicle
Posterior longitudinal ligament
Vertebral artery
Vertebral body
Annulus fibrosus
Nucleus pulposus
Intervertebral cartilage (disc)
Anterior longitudinal ligament

Typical Vertebrae (Superior View)

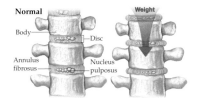

Cervical vertebra
Thoracic vertebra
Lumbar vertebra

The Spinal Column (Lateral View)

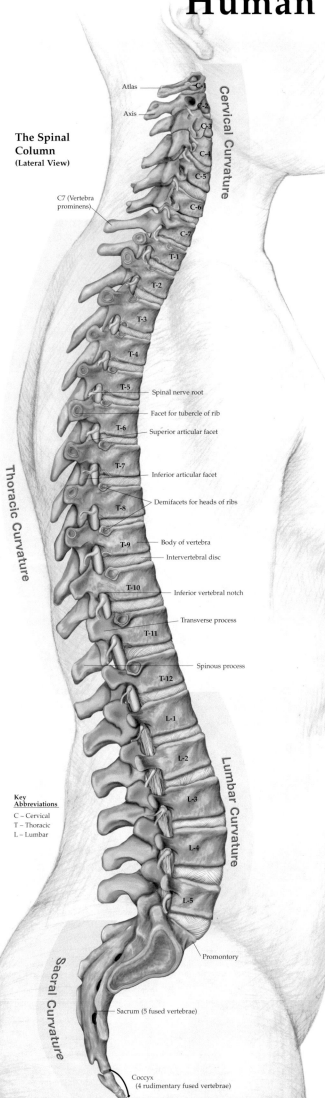

Atlas
Axis
C-1
C-2
C-3
C-4
C-5
C-6
C-7
C7 (Vertebra prominens)
Cervical Curvature
T-1
T-2
T-3
T-4
T-5
Spinal nerve root
Facet for tubercle of rib
T-6
Superior articular facet
T-7
Inferior articular facet
T-8
Demifacets for heads of ribs
T-9
Body of vertebra
Intervertebral disc
T-10
Inferior vertebral notch
Transverse process
T-11
Spinous process
T-12
Thoracic Curvature
L-1
L-2
L-3
L-4
L-5
Lumbar Curvature
Promontory
Sacrum (5 fused vertebrae)
Sacral Curvature
Coccyx (4 rudimentary fused vertebrae)

Key Abbreviations
C – Cervical
T – Thoracic
L – Lumbar

Structural Features of an Intervertebral Disc (Schematic)

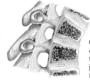

Nucleus pulposus
Annulus fibrosus

Note alternating obliquity of collagen fibrils.

The nucleus pulposus is the central gelatinous cushioning part of the intervertebral disc enclosed in several layers of cartilaginous laminae. The nucleus pulposus becomes dehydrated with age.

Function of Intervertebral Discs

Normal
Weight
Body
Disc
Annulus fibrosus
Nucleus pulposus

The disc, which contains nucleus pulposus, functions to protect the vertebrae from pressure.

Pathology

Osteoporosis

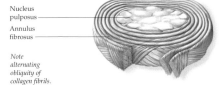

Osteoporosis develops when the body loses bone more quickly than it can make new bone. As a result, bones become less dense at the core and lose thickness at the surface. This increases the bones' susceptibility to fracture.

When osteoporosis involves the lumbar region, the vertebral bodies become markedly biconcave and the discs are ballooned.

Compression fractures * commonly occur at the thoracolumbar vertebral junction, resulting in wedge-shaped vertebrae.

* Fractures of laminae, pedicles, or transverse processes of the vertebrae are common.

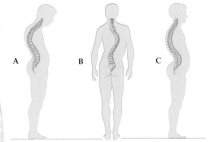

A   B   C

A. Hyperkyphosis
An excessive rounding of the thoracic vertebral column (humpback or hunchback).

B. Scoliosis
A curvature of the spine, often with twisting of the spinal column.

C. Hyperlordosis
A forward/anterior curvature of the cervical and lumbar (lower back) regions of the spine. In the lumbar region, it is also called "swayback."

Causes of Pain in the Back or Extremities

Shown below are other causes of pain that the examining physician should consider in making the diagnosis.

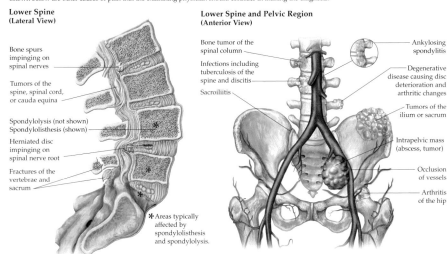

Lower Spine (Lateral View)

Bone spurs impinging on spinal nerves
Tumors of the spine, spinal cord, or cauda equina
Spondylolysis (not shown) Spondylolisthesis (shown)
Herniated disc impinging on spinal nerve root
Fractures of the vertebrae and sacrum

* Areas typically affected by spondylolisthesis and spondylolysis.

Lower Spine and Pelvic Region (Anterior View)

Bone tumor of the spinal column
Infections including tuberculosis of the spine and discitis
Sacroiliitis
Ankylosing spondylitis
Degenerative disease causing disc deterioration and arthritic changes
Tumors of the ilium or sacrum
Intrapelvic mass (abscess, tumor)
Occlusion of vessels
Arthritis of the hip

Understanding Osteoporosis

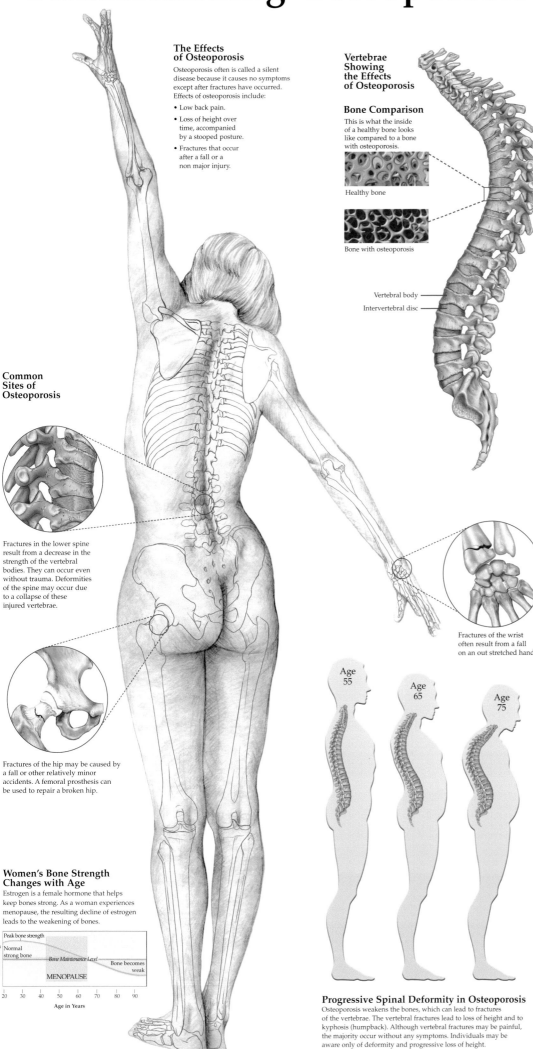

60

The Effects of Osteoporosis

Osteoporosis often is called a silent disease because it causes no symptoms except after fractures have occurred. Effects of osteoporosis include:

- Low back pain.
- Loss of height over time, accompanied by a stooped posture.
- Fractures that occur after a fall or a non major injury.

Common Sites of Osteoporosis

Fractures in the lower spine result from a decrease in the strength of the vertebral bodies. They can occur even without trauma. Deformities of the spine may occur due to a collapse of these injured vertebrae.

Fractures of the hip may be caused by a fall or other relatively minor accidents. A femoral prosthesis can be used to repair a broken hip.

Fractures of the wrist often result from a fall on an out stretched hand.

Vertebrae Showing the Effects of Osteoporosis

Bone Comparison

This is what the inside of a healthy bone looks like compared to a bone with osteoporosis.

Healthy bone

Bone with osteoporosis

Vertebral body

Intervertebral disc

What Is Osteoporosis?

Osteoporosis develops when the body loses bone more quickly than it can make it. As a result, bones become less dense at the core and lose thickness at the surface. This increases the bones' susceptibility to fracture.

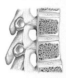

Normal vertebrae   Mild osteoporosis   Severe osteoporosis

Risk Factors

With aging, everyone has some bone loss. Certain people are likely to have even greater bone loss. Here are some factors that create a higher risk.

- Female (women are at a higher risk for osteoporosis than men are).
- Advancing age (over 50 years old).
- Family history of osteoporosis.
- Inactive lifestyle.
- Thin or small body size.
- Low-calcium diet.
- Vitamin D deficiency.
- Went through menopause at an early age.
- Smoking.
- Frequent alcohol use.
- Other medical conditions, such as chronic kidney failure, intestinal disease, and overactive thyroid.
- Certain medications, such as glucocorticoids (which are used to control diseases such as arthritis and asthma), some anti-seizure drugs, certain sleeping pills, some hormones used to treat endometriosis, and some cancer drugs.
- Race—Caucasians and Asians have a higher risk of developing osteoporosis.

Prevention and Treatment

Strategies to reduce the chances of developing osteoporosis include:

- Good eating and exercise habits, ideally from early in life. Building strong bones at a young age will lessen the effect of the natural bone loss that begins to occur around age 30.
- Adequate intake of calcium rich foods.
- Regular exercise, including weight-bearing activities, which put stress on the bones.
- Not smoking.
- Limit alcohol use.
- Consulting with a physician to find out if you should have a bone mineral density test.

How Much Calcium Do I Need?

Children 800 mg (4-8 years)

Teenagers 1,300 mg (9-18 years)

Adults 1,000 mg (19-50)

Adults 1,200 mg (51 or older)

Women 1,200 mg (pregnant or nursing)

Women 1,200-1,500 mg (postmenopausal)

Drug therapy can be used to prevent and to treat osteoporosis. The following drugs have been approved by the U.S. Food and Drug Administration to preserve or increase bone mass and maintain bone quality to reduce the risk of fractures:

- Estrogen replacement therapy (ERT).*
- Hormone replacement therapy (HRT).*
- Biophosphonates.
- Selective estrogen receptor modulators (SERMs).
- Hormones to regulate calcium and bone metabolism.

Other methods to prevent and treat osteoporosis are being studied. Consult with your doctor to determine the best plan of treatment.

* Because of the non-bone-related effects of these drugs, their long-term use in managing osteoporosis must be carefully considered.

How Do I Know If I Have Low Bone Mass?

Bone density is a term that describes how solid your bones are. In order to determine your bone density and fracture risk for osteoporosis, a bone mineral density (BMD) test must be done. In general, the lower your bone density, the higher your risk for fracture. There are several different machines that measure bone density. All are painless, noninvasive, and safe. In many testing centers you don't even have to change into an examining robe.

Ask your doctor about this test if you think you are at risk for osteoporosis, if you are a woman around the age of menopause, or if you are a man or woman over age 65.

What's Your T-score?

Your T-score	What It Means
Above -1.0	Bone mass is about normal.
-1.0	Bone mass is about 10% below normal.
-1.5	Bone mass is about 15% below normal.
-2.0	Bone mass is about 20% below normal.
You are considered osteoporotic if your T-score is -2.5 or less.	

Your bone mineral density (BMD) is compared to two norms, "young normal" and "age-matched." Your T-score compares your BMD to the peak bone density of a 30-year-old healthy adult. Your fracture risk increases when your BMD falls below "young normal" levels.

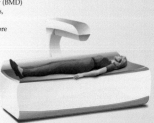

Women's Bone Strength Changes with Age

Estrogen is a female hormone that helps keep bones strong. As a woman experiences menopause, the resulting decline of estrogen leads to the weakening of bones.

Peak bone strength

Normal strong bone

Bone Maintenance Level

Bone becomes weak

MENOPAUSE

Bone Strength

20 30 40 50 60 70 80 90

Age in Years

Age 55

Age 65

Age 75

Progressive Spinal Deformity in Osteoporosis

Osteoporosis weakens the bones, which can lead to fractures of the vertebrae. The vertebral fractures lead to loss of height and to kyphosis (humpback). Although vertebral fractures may be painful, the majority occur without any symptoms. Individuals may be aware only of deformity and progressive loss of height.

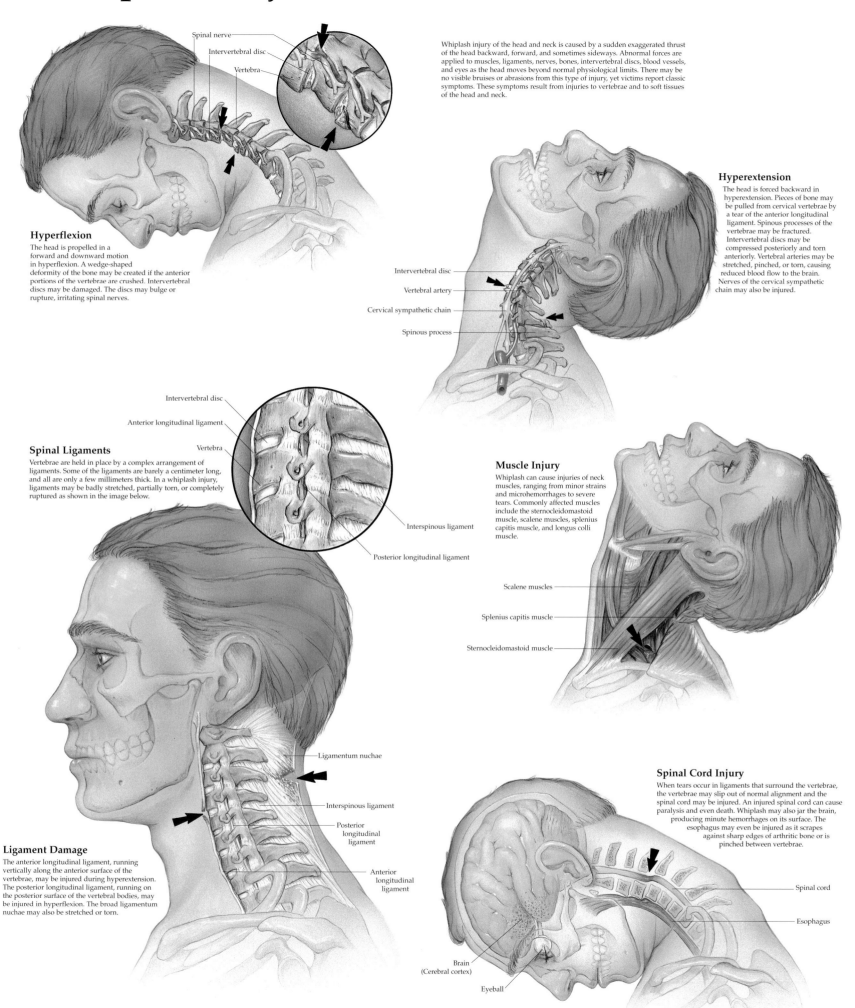

Whiplash injury of the head and neck is caused by a sudden exaggerated thrust of the head backward, forward, and sometimes sideways. Abnormal forces are applied to muscles, ligaments, nerves, bones, intervertebral discs, blood vessels, and eyes as the head moves beyond normal physiological limits. There may be no visible bruises or abrasions from this type of injury, yet victims report classic symptoms. These symptoms result from injuries to vertebrae and to soft tissues of the head and neck.

Spinal nerve
Intervertebral disc
Vertebra

Hyperflexion

The head is propelled in a forward and downward motion in hyperflexion. A wedge-shaped deformity of the bone may be created if the anterior portions of the vertebrae are crushed. Intervertebral discs may be damaged. The discs may bulge or rupture, irritating spinal nerves.

Hyperextension

The head is forced backward in hyperextension. Pieces of bone may be pulled from cervical vertebrae by a tear of the anterior longitudinal ligament. Spinous processes of the vertebrae may be fractured. Intervertebral discs may be compressed posteriorly and torn anteriorly. Vertebral arteries may be stretched, pinched, or torn, causing reduced blood flow to the brain. Nerves of the cervical sympathetic chain may also be injured.

Intervertebral disc
Vertebral artery
Cervical sympathetic chain
Spinous process

Spinal Ligaments

Vertebrae are held in place by a complex arrangement of ligaments. Some of the ligaments are barely a centimeter long, and all are only a few millimeters thick. In a whiplash injury, ligaments may be badly stretched, partially torn, or completely ruptured as shown in the image below.

Intervertebral disc
Anterior longitudinal ligament
Vertebra
Interspinous ligament
Posterior longitudinal ligament

Muscle Injury

Whiplash can cause injuries of neck muscles, ranging from minor strains and microhemorrhages to severe tears. Commonly affected muscles include the sternocleidomastoid muscle, scalene muscles, splenius capitis muscle, and longus colli muscle.

Scalene muscles
Splenius capitis muscle
Sternocleidomastoid muscle

Ligamentum nuchae
Interspinous ligament
Posterior longitudinal ligament
Anterior longitudinal ligament

Ligament Damage

The anterior longitudinal ligament, running vertically along the anterior surface of the vertebrae, may be injured during hyperextension. The posterior longitudinal ligament, running on the posterior surface of the vertebral bodies, may be injured in hyperflexion. The broad ligamentum nuchae may also be stretched or torn.

Spinal Cord Injury

When tears occur in ligaments that surround the vertebrae, the vertebrae may slip out of normal alignment and the spinal cord may be injured. An injured spinal cord can cause paralysis and even death. Whiplash may also jar the brain, producing minute hemorrhages on its surface. The esophagus may even be injured as it scrapes against sharp edges of arthritic bone or is pinched between vertebrae.

Spinal cord
Esophagus
Brain (Cerebral cortex)
Eyeball

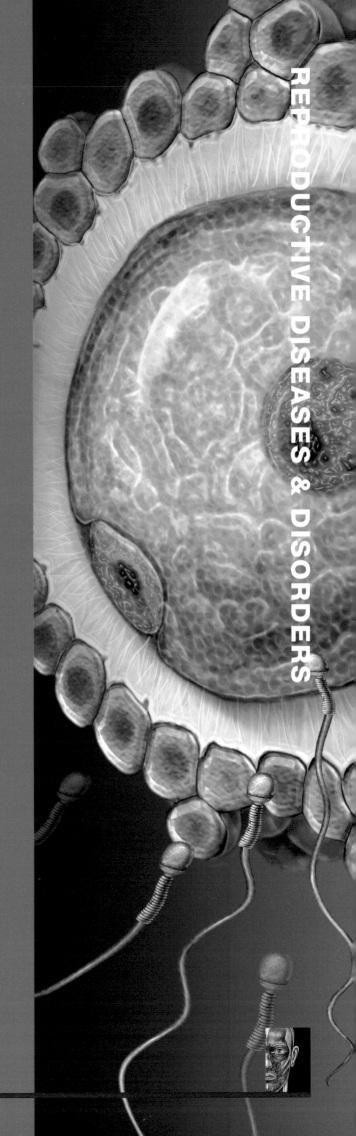

REPRODUCTIVE DISEASES & DISORDERS

• Benign Breast Disease • Common Gynecological Disorders • Infertility • Understanding Erectile Disfunction • The Prostate • Sexually Transmitted Infections (STIs) • Diseases of the Urinary Tract

63

Benign Breast Disease

What is Benign Breast Disease?

Certain types of non-cancerous conditions found in the breast are called **benign breast disease**. The most common types of benign breast disease are **benign breast tumors, breast inflammation and infection,** and **fibrocystic changes**. Normal hormonal changes probably are to blame for the growth of most benign breast changes.

There are two main types of breast tissue, **glandular** and **stromal**. The milk-producing lobules and their ducts are found in the glandular tissue. The stromal tissue is made up of fatty tissue and ligaments that support the breast.

Breast Self-Examination (BSE)

A BSE should be done at the same time every month. The best time to do a BSE is several days after your period ends. If you no longer menstruate (have periods), pick a certain day such as the first day of every month. Regular BSEs teach you how your breasts normally feel so you can more readily detect any changes.

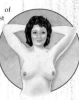

A. Stand in front of a mirror. Check each breast for anything unusual, such as dimpling, puckering, or scaliness of the skin. Check for discharge from the nipples. With your hands clasped behind your head, look for any change in the shape or contour of your breasts.

B. Press your hands firmly on your hips. Bend slightly toward the mirror as you pull your shoulders and elbows forward. Gently, squeeze each nipple and look for discharge.

C. Raise one arm. Use the pads of the fingers of your other hand to check each breast. Make sure also to check the underarm up to the collarbone and all of the way over the shoulder. Feel for any unusual lump or mass under the skin. Some women find this step easier to perform when standing in the shower using soap and water.

D. Repeat step C while lying on your back. Place one arm over your head and a pillow or rolled up towel under the same shoulder to raise the breast tissue and make it easier to check.

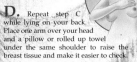

Circles   Edges   Lines

Feel the tissue by pressing your fingers in small, overlapping areas. Be sure to cover the entire breast. Take your time and follow a definite pattern such as **circles**, **edges**, or **lines**.

Symptoms

Healthcare providers often first find benign breast lumps during a clinical breast examination or mammogram. Breast self-examinations also are helpful in finding lumps. Symptoms of benign breast disease can include:

- Pain
- Tenderness
- Nipple pain or retraction
- Redness or scaliness of the breast skin or nipple
- Lump or swelling
- Skin irritation
- Tenderness (turning inward)
- A discharge other than milk

If you experience any of these symptoms, call your healthcare provider.

Treatment

Treatment for benign breast disease may include medications, changes in diet, or minor surgical procedures. Treatment will be determined based on:

- The patient's overall health and medical history
- Extent of the disease
- The patient's tolerance for specific medications, procedures, or therapies
- Outlook for the course of the disease
- The patient's opinion or preference

Diagnostic Procedures for a Detected Breast Abnormality

1) Medical History and Physical Exam
A healthcare provider performs a complete physical exam to locate the lump. He/she will note its texture, size, and relationship to the skin and chest muscles.

2) Nipple Discharge Evaluation
If there is nipple discharge, some of the fluid may be collected and examined. Most nipple discharge is benign.

3) Imaging Tests
- **Diagnostic mammography** is an X-ray examination of the breast that can show masses and tiny mineral deposits in the breast tissue.
- **Ultrasound** uses high-frequency sound waves to outline the breasts.

4) Biopsy
A biopsy is the removal and microscopic examination of a piece of tissue. Types of biopsies include:
- **Fine needle aspiration** uses a thin needle to remove fluid from a cyst or tissue from a mass.
- **Core needle biopsy** uses a somewhat larger needle with a special cutting edge. It removes a small sample of tissue.
- **A surgical biopsy** either removes the entire mass and a small area of surrounding tissue or removes only a small part of the mass.

(breast diagram labels)
Pectoralis major muscle
Stromal tissue: Fat
Glandular tissue: Gland lobules
Glandular tissue: Lactiferous duct
Nipple
Glandular tissue: Ampulla
Areola
External abdominal oblique muscle

Fibrocystic Breast Disease

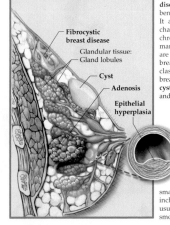

(diagram labels)
Fibrocystic breast disease
Glandular tissue: Gland lobules
Cyst
Adenosis
Epithelial hyperplasia

The term **fibrocystic breast disease** describes a variety of benign changes of the breast. It also is called fibrocystic change, cyclic disease, chronic cystic mastitis, or mammary dysplasia. There are several types of solitary breast lumps that can be classified as fibrocystic breast disease. These include **cysts, galactoceles, adenosis,** and **epithelial hyperplasia**.

Cysts
Cysts (fluid-filled sacs) found in the breast, often get bigger and become tender just before a menstrual period. They range in size from lumps that are too small to be felt to 1 to 2 inches in diameter. Cysts usually appear as movable, smooth, rounded lumps.

Galactoceles
Galactoceles look like cysts but instead they are filled with milk. They can occur in women who are pregnant or breast-feeding. Usually they appear as smooth, movable lumps, but on occasion, they can be hard or unmovable.

Adenosis
The excessive growth of lobule tissue is called adenosis. Since it can easily be mistaken for cancer, a biopsy is usually required. Women with adenosis do have a slight chance of getting breast cancer.

Epithelial Hyperplasia
An increase in the number of normal cells that line either the ducts or the lobules of the breast is called epithelial hyperplasia. Women with this condition have a greater chance of getting breast cancer.

Benign Breast Tumors

(diagram labels)
Fibroadenoma
Glandular tissue: Gland lobules
Intraductal papilloma
Glandular tissue: Lactiferous ducts
Nipple
Glandular tissue: Ampulla
Fat necrosis

Fibroadenomas
Fibroadenomas are common benign breast tumors. They range in size from microscopic to several inches in diameter. Often fibroadenomas stop growing or even shrink on their own without treatment.

Intraductal Papilloma
Intraductal papillomas are small, benign growths that most often develop in the large milk duct (lactiferous duct) near the nipple. They often cause bloody discharge.

Fat Necrosis
Fat necrosis is a benign condition in which fat cells die, usually after injury to the breast. Many times, scar tissue forms at the site of injury. Areas of fat necrosis sometimes form a saclike collection of greasy fluid called an oil cyst.

Granular Cell Tumors
Usually found in the mouth or skin, granular cell tumors are sometimes found in the breast. They are movable, firm lumps and measure between ½ inch and 1 inch in diameter. At first, they can be mistaken for breast cancer.

Phyllodes Tumors
A phyllodes (or phylloides) tumor is a rare type of breast tumor. It forms in the connective tissue of the breast. Usually benign, on rare occasions it can be cancerous and can spread.

Breast Infection and Inflammation

(diagram labels)
Mastitis
Mammary duct ectasia

Mastitis
Any infection or inflammation of the breast is called mastitis. Most commonly, it affects women who are breast-feeding. If the skin around the nipple cracks, bacteria can enter the breast, leading to infection. If not treated early enough, a collection of pus (abscess) can result and may need to be drained. Signs of mastitis usually include redness, heat, and pain in the breast.

Mammary Duct Ectasia
When the ducts leading to the nipple become swollen and then fill with fluid, infection and inflammation can result. This is called mammary duct ectasia. If is not treated, scar tissue can form, which may pull the nipple inward. Mammary duct ectasia can be painful and produces a thick, sticky discharge.

64

Common Gynecological Disorders

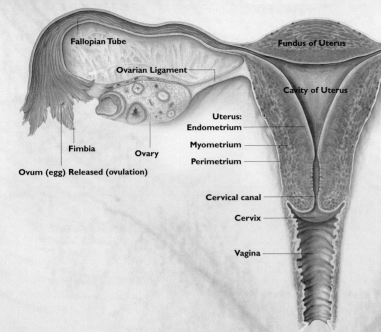

Fallopian Tube
Ovarian Ligament
Fundus of Uterus
Cavity of Uterus
Uterus:
Endometrium
Myometrium
Perimetrium
Fimbia
Ovary
Ovum (egg) Released (ovulation)
Cervical canal
Cervix
Vagina

NORMAL MENSTRUAL CYCLE

Monthly, from puberty through menopause, the menstrual cycle occurs in response to normal hormonal variations. The endometrial lining of the uterus thickens in preparation for the implantation of a fertilized egg. If pregnancy does not occur the lining of uterus is shed, resulting in a menstrual period. A normal menstrual cycle is 21 to 35 days.

ABNORMAL MENSTRUAL CYCLE

Abnormal vaginal bleeding is a flow of blood from the vagina that occurs either at the wrong time during a cycle or in inappropriate amounts brought on by various factors. Any history of abnormal vaginal bleeding warrants a visit to your doctor.

LACK OF MENSTRUAL BLEEDING -
Absence of menstruation (amenorrhea) may be due to anovulation, low estrogen levels, or a physical abnormality of the uterus. Causes include:

Asherman's Syndrome

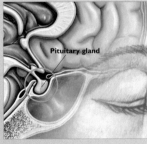

Band-like adhesions

Asherman's Syndrome is the presence of band-like adhesions that cross the lining of the uterus. This condition usually occurs after a surgical procedure such as dilatation and curettage (D&C).

Prolactinoma

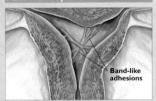

Pituitary gland

A prolactinoma is a benign (noncancerous) tumor of the pituitary gland that causes excess secretion of the prolactin hormone.

IRREGULAR BLEEDING -
Menstrual bleeding that is not regular or predictable is classified as irregular. Irregular bleeding tends to be anovulatory (ovulation does not occur) because the normal cyclic hormonal changes are inconsistent interfering with ovulation. Women may experience lack of menstruation or unpredictable bleeding. Causes include:

Polycystic Ovary Syndrome (PCOS)

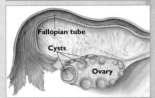

Fallopian tube
Cysts
Ovary

Rather than releasing an egg every month, women with polycystic ovary syndrome (PCOS) have ovarian follicles that develop into small cysts and remain in the ovary.

Eating Disorders & Extreme Exercise

Eating disorders or long, strenuous exercise programs may cause anovulatory cycles. These women may experience absence of menstruation or irregular menstrual cycles and may also be at risk for osteoporosis.

Medications

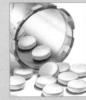

Many medications, including certain psychiatric and anti-seizure drugs, can cause anovulation and irregular bleeding. Hormones found in oral contraceptives or hormone therapy can cause abnormal bleeding as a side effect.

Vaginal & Uterine Atrophy (with menopause)

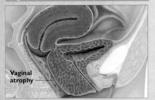

Vaginal atrophy

Vaginal and uterine atrophy can result in vaginal bleeding. Similarly, postmenopausal bleeding can be associated with endometrial hyperplasia and uterine cancer.

Hormonal Imbalances

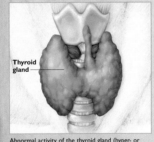

Thyroid gland

Abnormal activity of the thyroid gland (hyper- or hypothyroidism) can affect ovulation. Hyperprolactinemia (abnormally high level of the hormone prolactin) can also block ovulation.

REGULAR HEAVY BLEEDING -
Menstrual bleeding that is regular (monthly and predictable) and heavy or regular with bleeding in between periods (spotting) may be due to conditions that distort the uterine cavity or the body of the uterus. These conditions include benign tumors and growths. If bleeding is regular, it is likely that cyclic hormonal changes are also regular and that ovulation is occurring. Causes include:

Fibroids

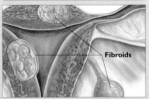

Fibroids

Fibroids are benign tumors of the muscle and connective tissue that develop within or are attached to the wall of the uterus; these may also cause painful periods.

Cervical Lesions

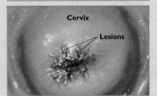

Cervix
Lesions

Cervical lesions are caused by the human papilloma virus (HPV). If left untreated they may progress to cervical cancer.

Von Willebrand's Disease

Von Willebrand's disease is an inherited bleeding disorder that may cause excessive bleeding during menstruation and/or surgery.

Polyps

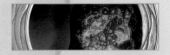

Polyps

Polyps are benign growths of the endometrium that can cause irregular bleeding and spotting.

Endometrial Hyperplasia

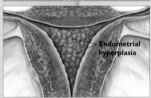

Endometrial hyperplasia

Endometrial hyperplasia is an abnormal overgrowth of the uterine lining (endometrium).

ABNORMAL VAGINAL DISCHARGE -
Normal vaginal discharge is a clear, white or off-white. The amounts are different for each individual and may change over time. Abnormal vaginal discharge has an unpleasant smell and can cause itching. The following conditions are associated with abnormal vaginal discharge:

Candidiasis (Yeast Infection)

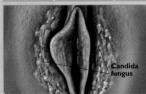

Candida fungus

Candidiasis of the vagina occurs when there is an overgrowth of the fungus called Candida. The discharge may resemble cottage cheese or may be watery, often has no smell, and usually causes vaginal itching.

Bacterial Vaginitis

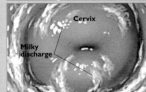

Cervix
Milky discharge

The most common vaginal infection occurring in women of reproductive age, bacterial vaginitis occurs when there is an overgrowth of bacteria. There is usually a thin, milky discharge with a fishy odor that may be more noticeable after sexual intercourse.

Trichomoniasis Vaginitis

Cervix
Microscopic view of parasite
Vaginal discharge

Trichomonas is a parasite that is generally spread through sexual contact. This infection may be asymptomatic (presenting no symptoms) but is generally associated with vaginal discharge, odor, and burning with urination.

Chlamydia and Gonorrhea

Chlamydia is a bacterial disease that is usually spread through sexual contact. This infection may be asymptomatic, but may be associated with an abnormal vaginal discharge or burning sensation when urinating. If the infection is left untreated and involves the fallopian tubes, it could cause pelvic inflammatory disease (PID) and infertility.

* Common sites for Chlamydia and Gonorrhea

Gonorrhea is a sexually transmitted infection disease caused by a bacterium that can infect the genital tract, the mouth, and the rectum. It is usually spread through sexual contact. Early symptoms can include bleeding during intercourse, painful/burning urination, and/or yellow or bloody vaginal discharge.

GYNECOLOGICAL/PELVIC PAIN -
Pain related to the pelvic and gynecological organs is a common symptom for many women. Pain can be caused by a variety of conditions. When experiencing pain, it is important to try to characterize the type of pain (crampy, sharp, etc.), the duration, and its relation to your menstrual cycle. This will help your health care provider to determine the cause of the pain.

Ovarian Cysts

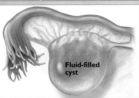

Fluid-filled cyst

Ovarian cysts range in size and the symptoms that they produce. Symptoms can range from asymptomatic, to dull ache/pressure, to pain. Some women may experience pain during intercourse.

Pelvic Inflammatory Disease (PID) & Pelvic Adhesions

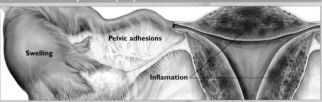

Swelling
Pelvic adhesions
Inflamation

Pelvic inflammatory disease (PID) is a general term that refers to infection of the uterus, fallopian tubes and other reproductive organs. Pelvic adhesions can occur following surgery or a pelvic infection. Depending upon their location, they can be the cause of pelvic pain.

Endometriosis

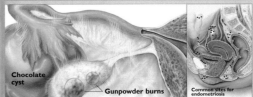

Chocolate cyst
Gunpowder burns
Common sites for endometriosis

Endometriosis occurs when the endometrium (the lining of the uterus) grows outside of the uterus. Pain symptoms can occur before and during periods and during or after intercourse.

Adenomyosis

Edenomyosis

Adenomyosis occurs when endometrial cells grow within the wall of the uterus. This can cause heavy and painful menstrual cycles.

©2008 Wolters Kluwer | Lippincott Williams & Wilkins I Published by Anatomical Chart Company, Skokie, IL

65

Infertility

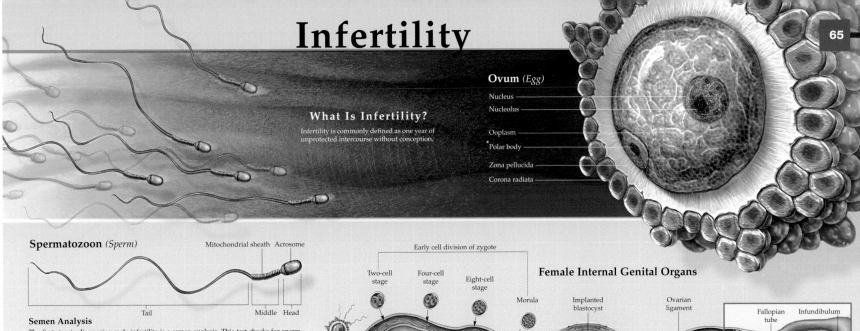

What Is Infertility?

Infertility is commonly defined as one year of unprotected intercourse without conception.

Ovum (*Egg*)

- Nucleus
- Nucleolus
- Ooplasm
- Polar body
- Zona pellucida
- Corona radiata

Spermatozoon (*Sperm*)

- Mitochondrial sheath
- Acrosome
- Tail
- Middle
- Head

Semen Analysis

The first step in diagnosing male infertility is a semen analysis. This test checks for sperm motility (movement), sperm morphology (shape and structure), and sperm count.

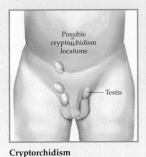

Possible cryptorchidism locations
- Testis

Cryptorchidism

Cryptorchidism is the failure of one or both testes to descend into the scrotum. In this congenital disorder, the testes remain in the abdomen or inguinal canal or at the external inguinal ring. Although this condition may be bilateral, it more commonly affects the right testis. True undescended testes remain along the path of normal descent.

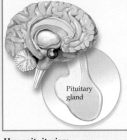

Pituitary gland

Hypopituitarism

The pituitary gland in the brain produces follicle stimulating hormone (FSH) and luteinizing hormone (LH). Both of these hormones act on the testes and are necessary for normal sperm production. A deficiency in the production of these hormones may cause abnormal sperm production.

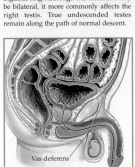

Vas deferens

Obstruction

Obstruction or absence of the vas deferens is a rare cause of infertility. The vas deferens carries the sperm from the testis through to the penis. If this structure is blocked or absent, sperm may be prevented from reaching the ejaculatory duct.

Varicocele

Varicocele

Varicocele is a mass of dilated and tortuous varicose veins in the spermatic cord. Blood pools in the plexus of veins rather than flowing into the venous system. Inadequate blood flow through the testis may affect sperm production and may lead to testicular atrophy.

Female Internal Genital Organs

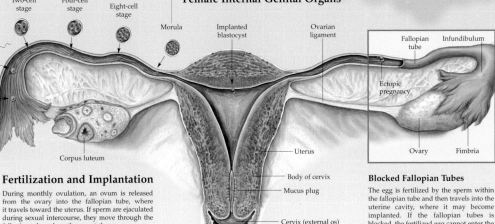

Early cell division of zygote
- Two-cell stage
- Four-cell stage
- Eight-cell stage
- Morula
- Implanted blastocyst
- Ovarian ligament
- Fertilization
- Ovum
- Corpus luteum
- Uterus
- Body of cervix
- Mucus plug
- Cervix (external os)
- Vagina
- Fallopian tube
- Infundibulum
- Ectopic pregnancy
- Ovary
- Fimbria

Fertilization and Implantation

During monthly ovulation, an ovum is released from the ovary into the fallopian tube, where it travels toward the uterus. If sperm are ejaculated during sexual intercourse, they move through the fallopian tube, where they meet the ovum.

If a sperm penetrates the ovum, fertilization occurs, and the ovum becomes a zygote. The zygote continues to travel toward the uterus, dividing many times until it becomes a blastocyst. There it implants in the uterine lining and in a normal pregnancy, continues to develop over the next nine months.

Blocked Fallopian Tubes

The egg is fertilized by the sperm within the fallopian tube and then travels into the uterine cavity, where it may become implanted. If the fallopian tubes is blocked, the fertilized egg cannot enter the uterus. Sometimes, a fertilized egg implants within the fallopian tube causing an ectopic (outside the uterus) pregnancy.

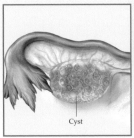

Cyst

Polycystic Ovarian Syndrome

Polycystic ovarian syndrome (PCOS) is associated with infrequent and irregular ovulation and multiple, small ovarian cysts. Some women with PCOS may also be overweight, have increased acne and hair growth, and are at risk for developing diabetes and uterine lining abnormalities.

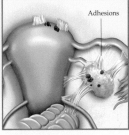

Adhesions

Pelvic Adhesions

The fallopian tube must be able to move freely in order to engulf the ovum (egg) after release from the ovary. Pelvic adhesions from previous infection, surgery, or endometriosis can interfere with the fallopian tube's mobility. The scar tissue can also affect the ovaries.

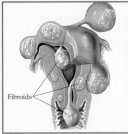

Fibroids

Intrauterine Fibroids

Fibroids are benign tumors of the uterus. Large submucosal fibroids can protrude into the uterine cavity and interfere with proper implantation of a fertilized egg. Fibroids can also block the opening of the fallopian tubes into the uterus and prevent a fertilized egg from entering the uterine cavity.

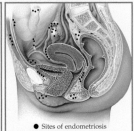

● Sites of endometriosis

Endometriosis

Endometriosis occurs when the tissue that normally lines the uterus grows outside it and in other areas of the body. It can cause scar tissue, pain, and infertility. In some cases the infertility may be attributed to the scar tissue, but there may also be an immunologic component.

Common Causes of Infertility

MALE

Abnormal sperm factors: If there is an abnormality in the semen analysis, further referral to a urologist may be needed. The World Health Organization (WHO) has published rough guidelines for normal semen analysis values.

Pre-testicular factors:
- Hypopituitarism – not enough pituitary hormones
- Hyperprolactinemia – too much prolactin hormone
- Hypothalamic dysfunction

Testicular factors:
- Certain drugs – can depress sperm quantity and quality
- Chemotherapy/radiation – may affect sperm count
- Testicular dysgenesis – failure of testes to form properly
- Cryptorchidism – failure of the testes to descend into the scrotum

Post-testicular factors:
- Obstruction of the vas deferens
- Varicocele – dilated and tortuous veins in the spermatic cord
- Retrograde ejaculation – sperm are deposited into the bladder following ejaculation. This can occur as a result of diabetes or neurologic disease, or occasionally following removal of the prostate gland
- Coital dysfunction - inability to ejaculate

Infertility Percentage Chart

The pie chart depicts the approximate distribution of the common causes of infertility among couples.

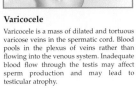

- Male problems — 35%
- Tubal and pelvic pathology (Female) — 35%
- Unusual problems (Either) — 5%
- Unexplained infertility (Either) — 10%
- Ovulatory dysfunction (Female) — 15%

FEMALE

Ovulatory dysfunction factors: The woman fails to ovulate or ovulates irregularly. Causes includes:
- Polycystic ovarian syndrome (PCOS)
- Age greater than 35 (increases the chance of decreased ovulation)
- Hyperprolactinemia – too much prolactin hormone
- Excessive exercise or dieting
- Drug or alcohol abuse
- Obesity

Tubal and pelvic pathology factors: Problems with fallopian tubes and ovaries, including:
- Pelvic adhesions – scar tissue affecting the fallopian tubes and ovaries
- Hydrosalpinx – fluid in the fallopian tubes
- Blocked fallopian tubes
- Endometriosis

Unusual problems, anatomic abnormalities, thyroid disease factors:
- Cervical factors like abnormal cervical mucus or prior cervical surgery
- Intrauterine fibroids or congenital abnormalities
- Immunologic antibody mediated sperm damage
- Hyper- or hypothyroidism
- Intrauterine adhesions

Unexplained infertility factors: Sometimes fertility test results are normal. Although there is probably a cause, it cannot be diagnosed with routine tests.

What Is Erectile Dysfunction?

Erectile dysfunction (*impotence*) is the persistent inability to obtain and maintain an erection sufficient for intercourse. Some men may experience complete erectile dysfunction, while others may achieve partial or brief erections. It is estimated 18 million to 30 million men in the United States are affected. Erectile dysfunction affects all age groups but increases in frequency with age.

What Causes Erectile Dysfunction?

A variety of medical conditions, the use of certain medicines and psychological problems may cause erectile dysfunction.

• Blood vessel (*vascular*) disease
Problems with the blood vessels that carry blood to the penis can reduce blood flow enough to impede erection. **Atherosclerosis** (*hardening of the arteries*) is the most common cause. **Cardiovascular disease**, **hypertension** (*high blood pressure*) and hypercholesterolemia (*high blood cholesterol*) can worsen the condition.

• Diabetes
Diabetes is a common cause of erectile dysfunction because diabetes can cause changes in blood flow through narrowing of the arteries or damage to nerve endings in the penis.

• Neurologic disease
Brain, spinal cord or **nerve injuries** (*especially to the nerves leaving the spinal cord, called the cauda equina*), as well as neurological diseases such as Alzheimer's disease, **stroke**, multiple sclerosis and Parkinson's disease can lead to erectile dysfunction.

• Hormone imbalance
Hormone imbalance, such as insufficient testosterone, causes only a small percentage of cases of erectile dysfunction. Testosterone is not directly involved in the vascular and neurologic events associated with penile erection.

• Pelvic surgery, trauma or radiation
Surgery, trauma or radiation to the prostate, bladder, rectum or colon can cause damage to the nerves or blood vessels in the surrounding area. Damage to pelvic nerves or arteries can result in erectile dysfunction.

• Psychological problems
Depression, anxiety, stress, low self-esteem and other mental conditions may lead to erectile dysfunction.

• Alcohol and drugs
Alcoholism and drug abuse are associated with erectile dysfunction, as is the use of certain **prescription drugs**. Medicines used to treat high blood pressure, heart disease, depression, psychosis and heartburn are among the most common medicines that interfere with the ability to have an erection.

• Chronic tobacco use
Smoking has been shown to affect the arteries in the penis, thus reducing blood flow necessary to maintain an erection.

How Is Erectile Dysfunction Treated?

The treatment depends on the cause of the erectile dysfunction. Behavior changes such as eliminating alcohol and drug abuse, cessation of smoking and reducing stress may improve erectile function.

Treatments include:

• Oral medication
Oral medication works directly on the blood vessels, causing the arteries to the penis to expand. It will cause an erection only when the man is sexually aroused.
Side effects: headaches, facial flushing, backache, upset stomach, bluish tinge to vision.

• Intraurethral pellets
The patient uses an applicator to insert a small pellet of medication into the opening at the end of the penis (*the urethra*). The medication causes blood vessels to relax, so the penis fills with blood and becomes erect.
Side effects: pain, burning sensation.

• Vacuum therapy
A cylinder is placed over the penis. By withdrawing air, a vacuum is created, mechanically enhancing the flow of blood into the penis. A rubber ring is placed at the base of the erect penis to trap the blood and maintain the erection.
Side effects: bruising, pain, diminished ejaculation.

• Penile injections
The patient uses a small needle to inject a powerful muscle relaxant into the base of the penis. The relaxation of muscle tissue allows blood to flow into the erectile tissues in the penis, creating an erection.
Side effects: pain, scarring, bleeding and rarely, prolonged erection.

• Penile implants
This requires a surgical intervention. Two inflatable balloons are implanted in the penis, as well as a pump into the scrotum and a reservoir near the bladder. When the pump is inflated, fluid from the reservoir flows into the inflatable balloons, creating an erection.
Side effects: infection, pain or malfunction.

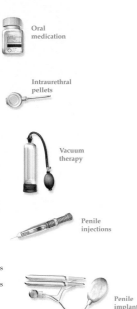

Atherosclerosis

Cardiovascular disease

Hypertension

Diabetes

Nerve injuries

Stroke

Alcohol and drugs

Smoking

Oral medication

Intraurethral pellets

Vacuum therapy

Penile injections

Penile implants

Male Reproductive Anatomy

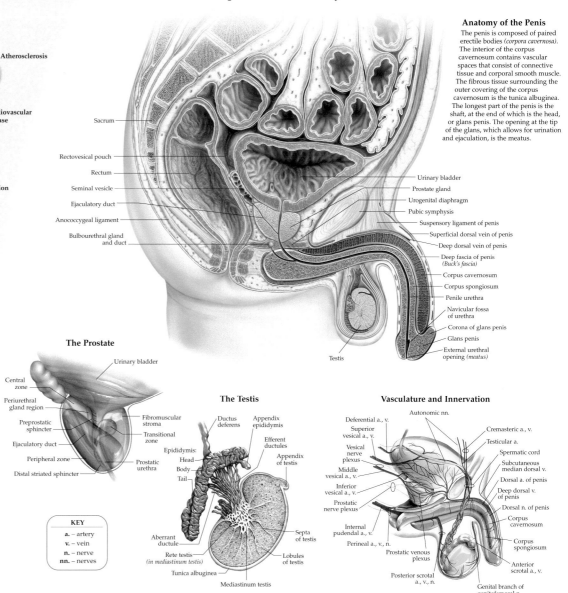

Anatomy of the Penis
The penis is composed of paired erectile bodies (*corpora cavernosa*). The interior of the corpus cavernosum contains vascular spaces that consist of connective tissue and corporal smooth muscle. The fibrous tissue surrounding the outer covering of the corpus cavernosum is the tunica albuginea. The longest part of the penis is the shaft, at the end of which is the head, or glans penis. The opening at the tip of the glans, which allows for urination and ejaculation, is the meatus.

Sacrum
Rectovesical pouch
Rectum
Seminal vesicle
Ejaculatory duct
Anococcygeal ligament
Bulbourethral gland and duct
Urinary bladder
Prostate gland
Urogenital diaphragm
Pubic symphysis
Suspensory ligament of penis
Superficial dorsal vein of penis
Deep dorsal vein of penis
Deep fascia of penis (*Buck's fascia*)
Corpus cavernosum
Corpus spongiosum
Penile urethra
Navicular fossa of urethra
Corona of glans penis
Glans penis
External urethral opening (*meatus*)
Testis

The Prostate
Urinary bladder
Central zone
Periurethral gland region
Preprostatic sphincter
Ejaculatory duct
Peripheral zone
Distal striated sphincter
Fibromuscular stroma
Transitional zone
Prostatic urethra

The Testis
Ductus deferens
Appendix epididymis
Efferent ductules
Appendix of testis
Epididymis: Head, Body, Tail
Aberrant ductule
Rete testis (*in mediastinum testis*)
Tunica albuginea
Mediastinum testis
Septa of testis
Lobules of testis

KEY
a. – artery
v. – vein
n. – nerve
nn. – nerves

Vasculature and Innervation
Autonomic nn.
Deferential a., v.
Superior vesical a., v.
Vesical nerve plexus
Middle vesical a., v.
Inferior vesical a., v.
Prostatic nerve plexus
Internal pudendal a., v.
Perineal a., v., n.
Prostatic venous plexus
Posterior scrotal a., v., n.
Cremasteric a., v.
Testicular a.
Spermatic cord
Subcutaneous median dorsal v.
Dorsal a. of penis
Deep dorsal v. of penis
Dorsal n. of penis
Corpus cavernosum
Corpus spongiosum
Anterior scrotal a., v.
Genital branch of genitofemoral n.

Physiology of Erection

The physiological process of erection begins in the brain and involves the nervous and vascular systems. The erection process is initiated by chemical neurotransmitters in the brain such as epinephrine, acetylcholine and nitric oxide. Physical or psychological stimulation causes nerves to send signals to the vascular system to increase blood flow to the penis. The erectile tissues of the penis expand as a result of the increased blood flow and pressure. To maintain rigidity, blood must stay in the penis. The erectile tissues are enclosed by fibrous elastic sheaths that prevent blood from leaving the penis during erection. When stimulation ends, or following ejaculation, pressure in the penis decreases, blood is released and the penis resumes its normal shape.

Nerve Distribution

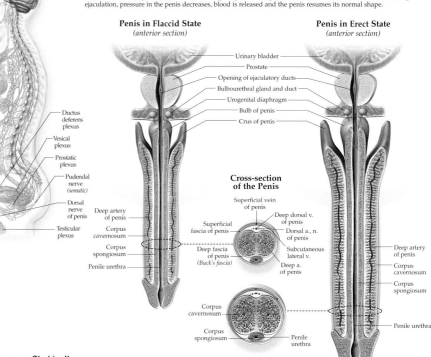

Brain
Ductus deferens plexus
Vesical plexus
Prostatic plexus
Pudendal nerve (*somatic*)
Dorsal nerve of penis
Testicular plexus

Penis in Flaccid State
(*anterior section*)

Penis in Erect State
(*anterior section*)

Urinary bladder
Prostate
Opening of ejaculatory ducts
Bulbourethral gland and duct
Urogenital diaphragm
Bulb of penis
Crus of penis

Cross-section of the Penis
Superficial vein of penis
Deep dorsal v. of penis
Dorsal a., n. of penis
Subcutaneous lateral v.
Deep a. of penis
Superficial fascia of penis
Deep fascia of penis (*Buck's fascia*)
Corpus cavernosum
Corpus spongiosum
Penile urethra

Deep artery of penis
Corpus cavernosum
Corpus spongiosum

Corpus cavernosum
Corpus spongiosum
Penile urethra

Deep artery of penis
Corpus cavernosum
Corpus spongiosum
Penile urethra

©2008 Wolters Kluwer Health | Lippincott Williams & Wilkins | Published by **Anatomical Chart Company, Skokie, IL**

The Prostate

Hormonal Influence on the Prostate

The prostate functions continuously, producing fluid which empties into the urethra. Hormones from the **pituitary gland** direct the **adrenal glands** and the **testes** to send chemical signals to the **prostate** to promote fluid production.

- Pituitary
- Adrenal gland
- Kidney
- Ureter
- Urinary bladder
- Prostate
- Testis

What is the Prostate?

The prostate is a gland consisting of fibrous, muscular and glandular tissue surrounding the urethra below the urinary bladder. Its function is to secrete prostatic fluid as a medium for semen, helping it to reach the female reproductive tract. Within the prostate, the urethra is joined by two ejaculatory ducts. During sexual activity, the prostate acts as a valve between the urinary and reproductive tracts. This enables semen to ejaculate without mixing with urine. Prostatic fluid is delivered by the contraction of muscles around gland tissue. Nerve and hormonal influences control the secretory and muscular functions of the prostate.

Normal Prostate (sagittal section)

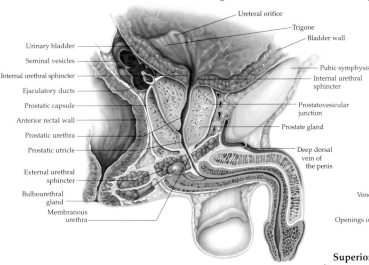

- Ureteral orifice
- Trigone
- Bladder wall
- Urinary bladder
- Seminal vesicles
- Internal urethral sphincter
- Ejaculatory ducts
- Prostatic capsule
- Anterior rectal wall
- Prostatic urethra
- Prostatic utricle
- External urethral sphincter
- Bulbourethral gland
- Membranous urethra
- Pubic symphysis
- Internal urethral sphincter
- Prostatovesicular junction
- Prostate gland
- Deep dorsal vein of the penis

Posterior View (dissected)

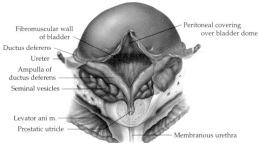

- Fibromuscular wall of bladder
- Ductus deferens
- Ureter
- Ampulla of ductus deferens
- Seminal vesicles
- Levator ani m.
- Prostatic utricle
- Peritoneal covering over bladder dome
- Membranous urethra

Anterior View with Exposed Prostatic Urethra

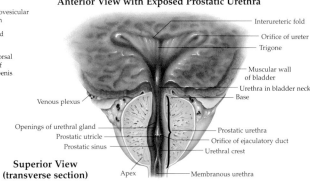

- Interureteric fold
- Orifice of ureter
- Trigone
- Muscular wall of bladder
- Urethra in bladder neck
- Base
- Venous plexus
- Openings of urethral gland
- Prostatic utricle
- Prostatic sinus
- Apex
- Prostatic urethra
- Orifice of ejaculatory duct
- Urethral crest
- Membranous urethra

Superior View (transverse section)

- Prostate glandular tissue lobes
- Prostatic urethra
- Prostatic utricle
- Ejaculatory ducts

Secretory gland with grape-shaped **acinus** end.

Vasculature and Innervation

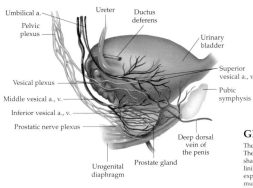

- Umbilical a.
- Pelvic plexus
- Ureter
- Ductus deferens
- Urinary bladder
- Superior vesical a., v.
- Vesical plexus
- Middle vesical a., v.
- Inferior vesical a., v.
- Prostatic nerve plexus
- Pubic symphysis
- Deep dorsal vein of the penis
- Urogenital diaphragm
- Prostate gland

Zones of the Prostate

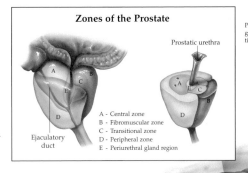

- Prostatic urethra
- Ejaculatory duct

A - Central zone
B - Fibromuscular zone
C - Transitional zone
D - Peripheral zone
E - Periurethral gland region

Glands of the Prostate

The prostate is mainly filled with secretory glands. These glands are made of many ducts with grape-shaped saccule ends or "acini". Secretory cells lining the ducts are stimulated by hormones to expel prostatic fluid. During sexual activity muscle contracts and secrete prostatic fluid. The basal cell, also found lining the ducts of the prostate, may be responsible for most types of prostatic hyperplasia as a result of uncontrolled prostatic tissue growth.

- **Secretory cells** are the most numerous in the gland and form the inner lining.
- Prostatic duct
- The **basal cell** is located below the lining surface and may function to rebuild prostatic tissue after infection or other damage.
- Fibromuscular stroma
- Ductal lumen
- Prostatic fluid

Benign Prostatic Hyperplasia (BPH)

Benign Prostatic Hyperplasia (BPH), is the most common type of tumor in mature men. It is a benign growth, which means it may enlarge but will not spread to other locations in the body. The tumor can cause discomfort and may grow to completely close the bladder neck, preventing urination. This condition occurs because the tumor usually grows in the transitional zone and periurethral gland region located at the prostate base near the bladder neck.

Early BPH:

Narrowing of the prostatic urethra causing difficulty in starting, maintaining, and stopping urination.

- Prostatic urethra

Prostatitis

Prostatitis is an uncomfortable condition in which the prostate becomes inflamed and swollen due to an infection. Prostatitis can make urinating painful.

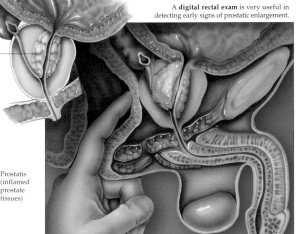

A **digital rectal exam** is very useful in detecting early signs of prostatic enlargement.

- Prostatis (inflamed prostate tissues)

Prostate Cancer

Prostate carcinoma is the most common malignant tumor in men. Unlike BPH, prostate cancer not only enlarges but also metastasizes (spreads) to other parts of the body through lymphatic and venous channels.

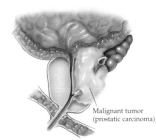

- Malignant tumor (prostatic carcinoma)

Pathways of Prostate Cancer Spread

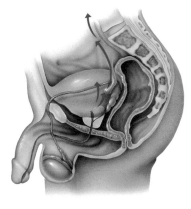

©2008 Wolters Kluwer Health | Lippincott Williams & Wilkins | Published by Anatomical Chart Company, Skokie, IL

What Are Sexually Transmitted Infections?

Sexually transmitted infections (STIs) are diseases you can get by having sex with someone who has an infection. There are more than 20 types of STIs, which can be spread during vaginal, oral, and anal sexual contact. STIs can be painful, and may have serious consequences (including death) if not treated. **Bacterial** STIs like gonorrhea and chlamydia are relatively easy to cure if treated early, but viral STIs, like genital herpes and the human immunodeficiency virus (HIV) cannot be cured. Other STIs such as trichomoniasis are caused by **protozoa** (single-celled organisms), and **parasites** are responsible for pubic lice and scabies.

Complications

Without treatment, sexually transmitted infections can lead to serious health problems— especially in women. In addition, STIs increase the risk of acquiring and transmitting HIV, the virus that causes AIDS. Some complications of STIs and the organs affected are listed below:

A **Brain and Nervous System** - Headaches, brain damage, meningitis (inflamed lining of the brain), stroke, neurological disorders (nervous system problems), psychiatric illness, spinal damage

B **Eyes** - Conjunctivitis, blindness

C **Mouth and Throat** - Thrush (infection of the oral tissues), pharyngitis (inflamed throat)

D **Lungs** - Peumocystis carinii (form of pneumonia common in people with reduced immunity)

E **Heart and Blood Vessels** - Aortic stenosis (narrowing of artery and/or valve of the heart), inflammation of the aorta, aneurysm (bulging) of the aorta, Kaposi's sarcoma (AIDS-related cancer affecting walls of certain lymphatic vessels)

F **Skin** - Rashes, itching, blisters, ulcers

G **Intestines** - Dysentery (inflammation of the intestine, with abdominal pain and frequent, watery stools)

H **Urinary System** - Cystitis (inflammation of the bladder), urinary tract infections, urethritis (inflammation of urethra)

I **Bones and Joints** - Arthritis, bone aches

Reproductive system complications include:

Male– Prostatitis (inflammation of the prostate gland), sterility, impotence, epididymitis (inflammation of the epididymis), urethral stricture

Female– Pelvic scarring, genital damage, cervical cancer, infertility, vulvovaginitis (inflammation of vulva and vagina), ectopic (tubal) pregnancy

Signs and Symptoms

The table below lists some of the most common symptoms of STIs. It is important to remember that many women and men who have an STI often do not experience any symptoms at all. If you are experiencing any of the symptoms listed below or if you believe you have an STI, talk to your health care provider as soon as possible.

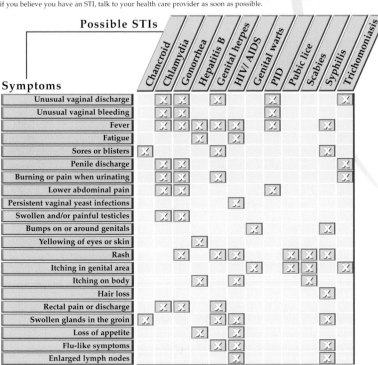

Possible STIs

Symptoms	Chancroid	Chlamydia	Gonorrhea	Hepatitis B	Genital herpes	HIV/AIDS	Genital warts	PID	Pubic lice	Scabies	Syphilis	Trichomoniasis
Unusual vaginal discharge		X	X		X							X
Unusual vaginal bleeding		X	X				X					
Fever	X	X	X	X	X	X		X				
Fatigue				X		X						
Sores or blisters	X				X							
Penile discharge		X	X									X
Burning or pain when urinating	X	X	X		X							X
Lower abdominal pain		X	X					X				
Persistent vaginal yeast infections						X						
Swollen and/or painful testicles	X	X										
Bumps on or around genitals							X		X	X		
Yellowing of eyes or skin				X								
Rash				X	X				X	X	X	
Itching in genital area							X		X	X		X
Itching on body				X		X				X		
Hair loss												X
Rectal pain or discharge	X	X	X								X	
Swollen glands in the groin	X				X						X	
Loss of appetite				X	X							
Flu-like symptoms				X		X						
Enlarged lymph nodes						X						X

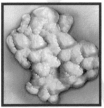

Genital Warts

Genital warts are painless growths found on or around the genital and anal areas. They are caused by the human papillomavirus (HPV). Despite treatment, genital warts cannot be cured and often recur. In women, infection with certain strains of HPV can increase the risk of developing cervical cancer.

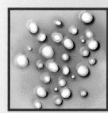

Genital Herpes

Genital herpes is a viral infection that causes painful sores on and around the genitals or anal area. It is easily spread and the disease tends to recur, especially in the first few years after initial infection. There is no cure, but there are medications that can help relieve symptoms.

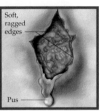

Soft, ragged edges

Pus

Chancroid

Chancroid (shan-kroid) is a bacterial infection that causes painful ulcers on the genitals. The chancroid ulcer can be difficult to distinguish from ulcers that are caused by genital herpes and syphilis. Symptoms usually appear within a week of exposure.

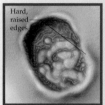

Hard, raised edges

Syphilis

Syphilis is a bacterial infection, that can damage organs over time if untreated. The first symptom of syphilis is an ulcer called a **chancre** (shan-ker). Left untreated, about one-third of cases will go onto the later, more damaging, stages.

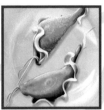

Trichomoniasis

One of the most common STIs, trichomoniasis (trick-oh-moh-nye-uh-sis) is a genital-tract infection caused by a protozoan (single-celled organism). This STI is usually transmitted through sexual intercourse, but a woman can also transmit the infection to her baby during childbirth.

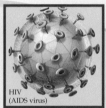

HIV (AIDS virus)

HIV/AIDS

HIV (human immuno-deficiency virus) infects and gradually destroys cells in the immune system. HIV severely weakens the body's response to infections and cancers. Eventually, AIDS (acquired immunodeficiency syndrome) is diagnosed. With AIDS, a variety of infections can overtake the body and eventually cause death.

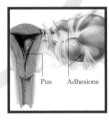

Pus   Adhesions

Pelvic Inflammatory Disease (PID)

PID is a term used to describe an infection of the uterus, fallopian tubes or ovaries. It is the most common, serious infection among young women. PID infection can cause scarring of the tissue inside the fallopian tubes, which can damage the tubes or block them completely. If untreated, PID can result in infertility, ectopic pregnancy, miscarriage, or chronic pain.

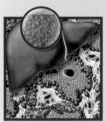

Hepatitis B

The liver disease Hepatitis B is caused by a virus carried in the blood, saliva, semen, and other body fluids of an infected person. It is spread through sexual contact and can be spread from a mother to her baby during childbirth or during breastfeeding. Recovery usually happens within six months, but in rare cases hepatitis B can lead to liver damage and an increased risk of liver cancer.

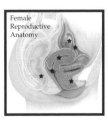

Pubic Lice

Pubic lice are tiny parasites that live in pubic hair and survive by feeding on human blood. They are most often spread by sexual activity, but in rare cases they can be spread through contact with infested clothing or bedding. It is unusual for pubic lice to cause any serious health problems, but the itching they cause can be very uncomfortable.

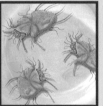

Scabies

Scabies is a parasitic skin infection caused by a tiny mite. Highly contagious, it is spread primarily through sexual contact, though it also can be spread through contact with skin, infested clothing, or bedding. Scabies causes intense itching, which often is worse at night.

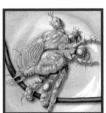

Female Reproductive Anatomy

Chlamydia

Chlamydia is a bacterial disease that produces an infection very similar to gonorrhea. Up to 50 percent of men, and 75 percent of women don't experience any symptoms. Complications for women are more serious than for men. In women chlamydia can cause irreversible damage, such as pelvic inflammatory disease and infertility.

★ = sites of infection for both chlamydia and gonorrhea

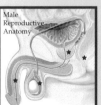

Male Reproductive Anatomy

Gonorrhea

Gonorrhea, is a curable STI which can infect the genital tract, the mouth, and the rectum. It is usually spread through sexual contact, but an infected woman can pass the disease to her baby during delivery. Often there are no symptoms. Untreated it can cause sterility in both sexes.

★ = sites of infection for both chlamydia and gonorrhea

Prevention and Treatment

The only way to eliminate the risk of acquiring an STI is to avoid sex *completely*. But there are several measures you can take to *reduce* your risk and to avoid transmitting STIs:

- Avoid sex with multiple partners.
- Use a condom.
- Get a Hepatitis B immunization (shot).
- Become familiar with the symptoms of STIs.
- Know your sexual partner's sexual history.

- Have regular checkups for STIs, even if you have no symptoms.
- Seek medical help immediately if any suspicious symptoms develop.

- If infected, tell any past or present partner(s) so that they may get treated.
- Avoid all sexual activity while being treated for an STI.

Most STIs are easily treated. The earlier a person seeks treatment, the less likely the disease will cause permanent physical damage, be spread to others, or be passed on from a mother to her newborn baby.

©2008 Wolters Kluwer | Lippincott Williams & Wilkins | Published by Anatomical Chart Company, Skokie, IL

Diseases of the Urinary Tract

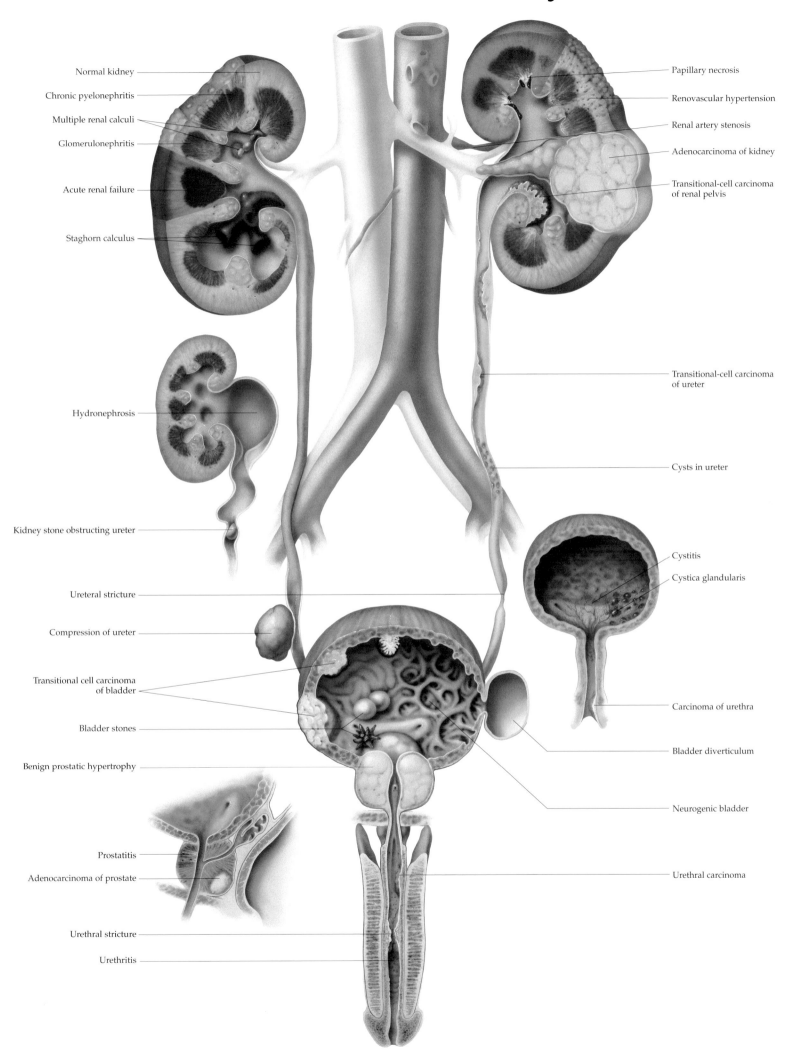

Normal kidney

Chronic pyelonephritis

Multiple renal calculi

Glomerulonephritis

Acute renal failure

Staghorn calculus

Hydronephrosis

Kidney stone obstructing ureter

Ureteral stricture

Compression of ureter

Transitional cell carcinoma of bladder

Bladder stones

Benign prostatic hypertrophy

Prostatitis

Adenocarcinoma of prostate

Urethral stricture

Urethritis

Papillary necrosis

Renovascular hypertension

Renal artery stenosis

Adenocarcinoma of kidney

Transitional-cell carcinoma of renal pelvis

Transitional-cell carcinoma of ureter

Cysts in ureter

Cystitis

Cystica glandularis

Carcinoma of urethra

Bladder diverticulum

Neurogenic bladder

Urethral carcinoma

©2008 Wolters Kluwer | Lippincott Williams & Wilkins I Published by Anatomical Chart Company, Skokie, IL
Health

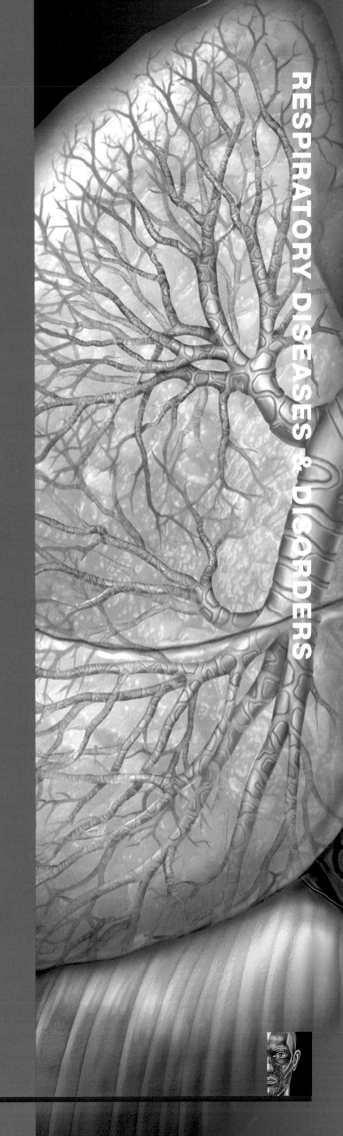

RESPIRATORY DISEASES & DISORDERS

71

Understanding Allergies

What Is An Allergy?

An allergy is an overreaction or hypersensitivity of the body's immune system to normally harmless substances, called allergens. An allergic reaction occurs when the body's immune system responds to an allergen as if the substance were disease causing. Subsequent exposures to this substance can result in physical symptoms that range from mild to life threatening.

Who Gets Allergies?

The tendency to develop allergies is thought to be inherited, because they commonly develop in those who have a family history of allergies. It is possible for anyone to develop allergies at any age. Environmental factors can make our immune systems overly sensitive. This could then trigger allergies in people with no family history or hasten the onset in those with a family history.

What Are Common Allergens?

Allergens can enter the body in a number of different ways, including inhaling, eating/drinking, injection (as with bee venom), and contact with the skin or eyes. Common allergens include pollen, mold, animal hair or dander, dust mites, certain medications (for example, penicillin), and certain foods (for example, peanuts, eggs, milk, wheat, and seafood).

Anaphylaxis: An Allergic Emergency

Anaphylaxis is a life-threatening reaction. The onset of this reaction may occur within seconds or minutes of exposure. Symptoms may include a red rash over most of the body. Skin becomes warm to the touch, intense tightening and swelling of the airways make breathing difficult, and there is a drop in blood pressure. Breathing can stop and the body may slip into shock. If medication is not administered quickly, heart failure and death can result within minutes in the most severe reactions. Allergens in insect venom and medications such as antibiotics are more likely to cause anaphylaxis than are any other allergens. Anaphylaxis is not a common reaction and can be controlled with prompt medication and the help of a physician.

Managing Allergies

The first step in managing allergies is to identify the type of reaction you are having, whether it is watery eyes, sneezing, or difficulty breathing. Second, try to identify the trigger or the situation that led to the symptoms. Ask yourself a few questions:

- *Where did the reaction occur?*
- *Inside or outside?*
- *Were you eating or drinking?*
- *Were there any animals or insects near you?*
- *Were you wearing any new clothing?*
- *Did you use a new soap or detergent?*

A physician can perform skin or blood allergy tests with a variety of common allergens. Once the allergen has been identified, manage your allergies by following some tips:

- *Avoid allergens when possible.*
- *Avoid tobacco smoke and other irritants.*
- *Use medication as prescribed.*
- *See a doctor regularly.*
- *Stay healthy.*

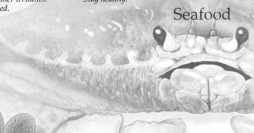

Seafood

Drugs

Mold

Peanuts

Pollen

Dander   Dust mites

©2008 Wolters Kluwer | Lippincott Williams & Wilkins
Health
Published by Anatomical Chart Company, Skokie, IL

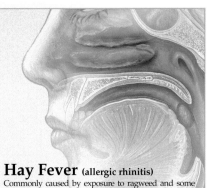

Hay Fever (allergic rhinitis)

Commonly caused by exposure to ragweed and some tree pollens. It affects the eyes and nose. Causes sneezing; runny nose; watery, itchy eyes; irritated, itchy throat; and sometimes, a stuffy, blocked nose.

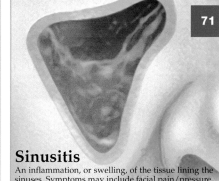

Sinusitis

An inflammation, or swelling, of the tissue lining the sinuses. Symptoms may include facial pain/pressure, a "stuffy head" (congestion), nasal stuffiness, nasal discharge, and loss of sense of smell.

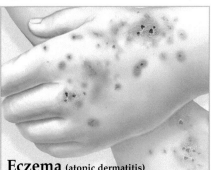

Eczema (atopic dermatitis)

A group of medical conditions that cause the skin to become inflamed or irritated. It causes itchy, red rashes of the skin characterized by lesions, scaling, and flaking.

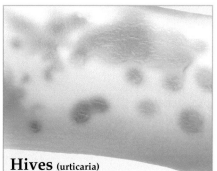

Hives (urticaria)

An outbreak of swollen, pale red bumps or patches (wheals) on the skin, as a result of the body's adverse reaction to certain allergens, or for unknown reasons.

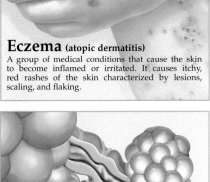

Asthma

Affects the respiratory system, causing coughing, wheezing, and chest tightness after exposure to an allergen. Common allergens that worsen asthma include plant pollens and dust mites.

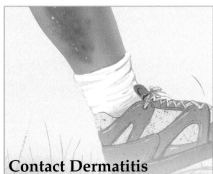

Contact Dermatitis

An inflammation of the skin caused by direct contact with an irritating or allergy-causing substance (such as poison ivy or latex gloves). It causes redness, itching, swelling, or rashes on the skin.

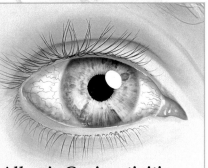

Allergic Conjunctivitis

An inflammation of the conjunctiva, the tissue that lines the eyeball and inside of the eyelid, associated with allergies. The eye becomes red, itchy, and watery.

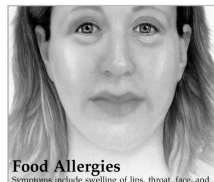

Food Allergies

Symptoms include swelling of lips, throat, face, and tongue; upset stomach; vomiting; abdominal cramps; hives; and skin rashes. Food allergies may be life threatening.

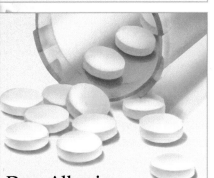

Drug Allergies

Certain medicines can trigger allergic reactions ranging from mild rashes to life-threatening symptoms, which can affect any tissue or organ in the body.

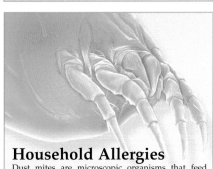

Household Allergies

Dust mites are microscopic organisms that feed on live and shed skin tissue. Mites are commonly found on pillows, mattresses, and upholstered furniture. Mite feces are responsible for a majority of the year-round types of allergies, and are a major cause of asthma.

72

Understanding Asthma

What Happens in an Asthma Attack?

What Is Asthma?

Asthma is a chronic disease of the lungs in which inflammation causes the airways to narrow, making breathing more difficult.

What Causes Asthma?

Although the actual cause of asthma is not known, many studies have shown that it may be due to a combination of factors. We do know that asthma is not contagious like the flu. We also know that people have a higher risk of developing asthma if a family member has had an asthma attack or if they live with people who smoke.

How Is Asthma Diagnosed?

There is no single or definitive test for asthma. It is diagnosed based on a review of the patient's medical history and those of his or her family. There are many tests your doctor may use to get more information about your condition. These include pulmonary function tests, allergy tests, blood tests, and chest and sinus x-rays.

A Smooth muscle tightens the airways.

Smooth muscle

Alveoli

B Sides of airways have become inflamed and swollen, making it harder for oxygen to get to alveoli.

Oxygen

C Excess mucus has formed inside the airways.

Sides of airways are thin to allow more space for oxygen to get to alveoli.

Oxygen

Bronchiole During an Asthma Attack

Healthy Bronchiole

Carbon dioxide exhaled **5**

Oxygen inhaled **1**

2

3

5 **4**

How Do the Lungs Work?

When you breathe, you draw in (inhale) fresh air and oxygen into your lungs and expel (exhale) stale air and carbon dioxide from your lungs.

1 The incoming air goes through a network of airways (bronchial tubes) that reach the lungs.

2 As the air moves through the lungs, the bronchial tubes become progressively smaller, like branches of a tree.

3 At the end of the smallest tubes are alveolar sacs, the site of gas exchange between the lungs and the circulatory system.

4 Oxygen enters the alveolar sacs, where it passes to the bloodstream and is then used by the body.

5 Carbon dioxide (waste product) from the bloodstream enters the alveolar sacs to be carried out of the lungs.

Monitoring Your Asthma by Zone

Green Zone	Yellow Zone	Red Zone
No asthma symptoms. Able to do usual activities and sleep without coughing, wheezing, or breathing difficulty.	There may be coughing, wheezing, and mild shortness of breath. Sleep and usual activities may be disturbed. May be more tired than usual.	Symptoms may include frequent, severe cough; severe shortness of breath; wheezing; trouble talking while walking; rapid breathing.
Action: Keep controlling/preventing your asthma symptoms. Continue to take your asthma medicines exactly as prescribed by your healthcare specialist, even if you have no symptoms and feel fine.	**Action:** Keep controlling your asthma symptoms and add your prescribed quick-relief medicine. Call to discuss the situation with your doctor or healthcare specialist.	**Action:** Go to an emergency room.

Symptoms of Asthma

Symptoms of asthma often vary from time to time in an individual. The severity of an asthma attack can increase rapidly, so it is important to treat your symptoms immediately once you recognize them.

Adult Symptoms
• Wheezing
• Chest tightness
• Coughing
• Difficulty breathing: shortness of breath

Childhood Symptoms
• Coughing at night or during sleep
• Diminished responsiveness
• Constant rattly cough
• Frequent chest colds
• Rapid breathing
• Weak cry
• Grunt when nursing or have difficulty feeding
• Chest might feel "funny"
• Unexplained irritability

Common Asthma Triggers

The airways in an asthmatic person are extremely sensitive to certain factors known as triggers. When stimulated by these triggers, the airways overreact with abnormal inflammation that leads to swelling, increased mucus secretion, and muscle contraction of the air passages. Examples of asthma triggers include:

• Pollution: cigarette smoke,* smog, strong odors from painting or cooking, scented products
• Allergens: animal dander, dust mites, cockroaches, pollen, mold
• Cold air or changes in weather
• Illness and infections
• Exercise
• Medications such as pain relievers
• Sulfites or other additives in food and beverages
• GERD (gastroesophageal reflux disease)

The proteins on dust mites are among the allergens that may trigger an asthma attack.

People can have trouble with one or more triggers. Your doctor can help you identify your asthma triggers and ways to avoid them.

*The risk of asthma is increased in children who are regularly exposed to cigarette smoke.

Management of Asthma

Asthma is a chronic disease that can be controlled to allow normal daily activities. By controlling your asthma every day, you can prevent serious symptoms and take part in all activities. If your asthma is not well controlled, you are likely to have symptoms that can make you miss school or work and keep you from doing other things you enjoy. Although there is no cure, here are some important prevention strategies:

• Recognize attacks early.
• Take medication as directed.
• Avoid tobacco smoke.
• Identify and avoid triggers.
• Talk with your doctor to find ways to improve your health.
• Get the influenza vaccination (flu shot) every year and a pneumococcal vaccination (pneumonia shot) every five years.

©2008 Wolters Kluwer Health | Lippincott Williams & Wilkins | Published by Anatomical Chart Company, Skokie, IL

73

Chronic Obstructive Pulmonary Disease (COPD)

Chronic Obstructive Pulmonary Disease (COPD)

Chronic obstructive pulmonary disease (COPD) is a term used to describe prolonged irreversible airflow obstruction that is mainly associated with emphysema and chronic bronchitis.

The most common chronic lung disease, COPD is a leading global health problem causing significant worldwide disability. COPD is the 4th leading cause of death and unfortunately its prevalence continues to rise. Early on, it does not always produce symptoms and causes only minimal disability in many patients. However, COPD tends to worsen with time.

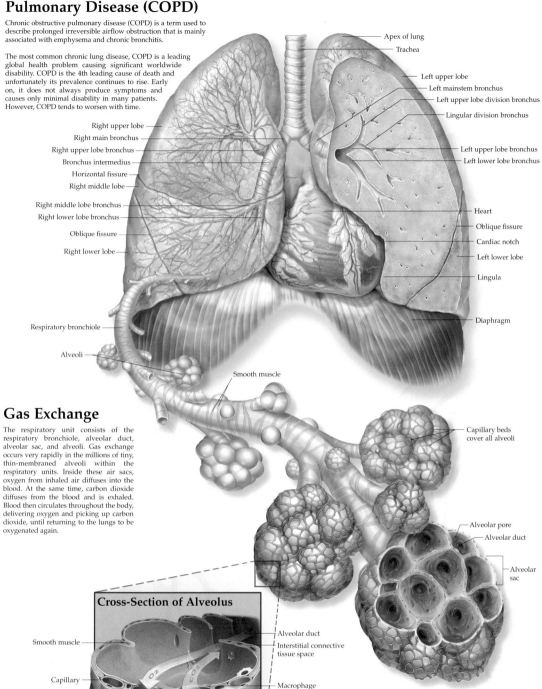

Labels (left lung): Right upper lobe; Right main bronchus; Right upper lobe bronchus; Bronchus intermedius; Horizontal fissure; Right middle lobe; Right middle lobe bronchus; Right lower lobe bronchus; Oblique fissure; Right lower lobe; Respiratory bronchiole; Alveoli

Labels (top/right): Apex of lung; Trachea; Left upper lobe; Left mainstem bronchus; Left upper lobe division bronchus; Lingular division bronchus; Left upper lobe bronchus; Left lower lobe bronchus; Heart; Oblique fissure; Cardiac notch; Left lower lobe; Lingula; Diaphragm

Smooth muscle

Gas Exchange

The respiratory unit consists of the respiratory bronchiole, alveolar duct, alveolar sac, and alveoli. Gas exchange occurs very rapidly in the millions of tiny, thin-membraned alveoli within the respiratory units. Inside these air sacs, oxygen from inhaled air diffuses into the blood. At the same time, carbon dioxide diffuses from the blood and is exhaled. Blood then circulates throughout the body, delivering oxygen and picking up carbon dioxide, until returning to the lungs to be oxygenated again.

Labels: Capillary beds cover all alveoli; Alveolar pore; Alveolar duct; Alveolar sac

Cross-Section of Alveolus

Labels: Smooth muscle; Capillary; Elastic fibers; Fibroblast; Alveolar cell: Type I pneumocyte, Type II pneumocyte; Alveolar duct; Interstitial connective tissue space; Macrophage; Basal lamina; Collagen fibril

Emphysema

In normal, healthy breathing, air moves in and out of the lungs to meet metabolic needs. Any change in airway size compromises the lungs' ability to circulate sufficient air.

In a patient with emphysema, recurrent pulmonary inflammation damages and eventually destroys the alveolar walls, causing them to break down and merge, creating large air spaces. This breakdown leaves the alveoli unable to recoil normally after expanding and results in bronchiolar collapse on exhalation. This traps air within the lungs, causing breathlessness.

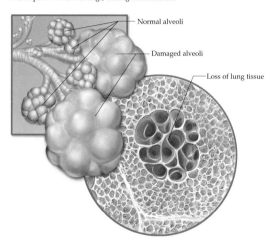

Labels: Normal alveoli; Damaged alveoli; Loss of lung tissue

Chronic Bronchitis

Chronic bronchitis is marked by excessive production of tracheobronchial mucus that is sufficient to cause a cough on most days for at least three months each year for two consecutive years.

In chronic bronchitis, irritants such as cigarette smoke inhaled for a prolonged period inflame the tracheobronchial tree. The inflammation leads to increased mucus production and a narrowed or blocked airway. As inflammation continues, the mucus-producing goblet cells undergo hypertrophy, as do the ciliated epithelial cells that line the respiratory tract. Hypersecretion from the goblet cells blocks the free movement of the cilia, which normally sweep dust, irritants, and mucus from the airways. As a result, the airway stays blocked, and mucus and debris accumulate in the respiratory tract.

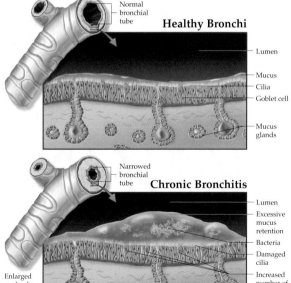

Healthy Bronchi

Labels: Normal bronchial tube; Lumen; Mucus; Cilia; Goblet cell; Mucus glands

Chronic Bronchitis

Labels: Narrowed bronchial tube; Lumen; Excessive mucus retention; Bacteria; Damaged cilia; Increased number of goblet cells; Enlarged mucous glands

Causes

Predisposing factors to COPD include:
- cigarette smoking
- recurrent or chronic respiratory infections
- air pollution
- allergies

Smoking is by far the most important of these factors. Smoking increases mucus production and impairs its removal from the airways, impedes the function of airway cells that digest disease-causing organisms, causes airway inflammation, destroys air sacs in the lungs, and leads to abnormal fibrous tissue growth in the bronchial tree.

Early inflammatory changes may reverse themselves if the person stops smoking before lung damage is extensive. Hereditary factors (such as deficiency of alpha-$_1$ antitrypsin) may also predispose a person to the development of COPD.

Symptoms

The typical COPD patient is a long-term smoker who has no symptoms until middle age, when his or her ability to exercise or do strenuous work starts to decline and a productive cough begins.

Subtle at first, these problems worsen as the patient ages and the disease progresses. Eventually, they cause difficulty breathing even on minimal exertion, frequent respiratory infections, oxygen deficiency in the blood, and abnormalities in pulmonary function.

When advanced, chronic bronchitis and emphysema may cause chest deformities, overwhelming disability, heart enlargement, severe respiratory failure, and death.

Diagnosis

Chest X-rays
Help to rule out pneumonia and lung cancer. They also show heart size. If the patient has emphysema, X-rays can pinpoint areas of damaged lung tissue.

Pulmonary Function Tests
Measure lung capacity and airway obstruction.

Arterial Blood Gas Analysis
Measures the amount of oxygen and carbon dioxide in the blood.

Electrocardiography
Measures the electric activity of the heart.

Sputum Analysis
Detects respiratory infection.

Treatment

Since the majority of cases of COPD are smoking-related, the patient should **avoid smoking**.

The main goal of treatment is to relieve symptoms and prevent complications. **Bronchodilators** can help alleviate bronchospasm and enhance mucociliary clearance of secretions. **Effective coughing, postural drainage, and chest physiotherapy** can help mobilize secretions.

In patients who require it, administration of low concentrations of **oxygen** helps relieve symptoms and prolongs life.

Antibiotics allow treatment of respiratory infections. **Pneumococcal vaccination and annual influenza vaccinations** are important in preventing complications.

Pulmonary rehabilitation improves quality of life, strength, and sense of well-being.

Diseases of the Lung

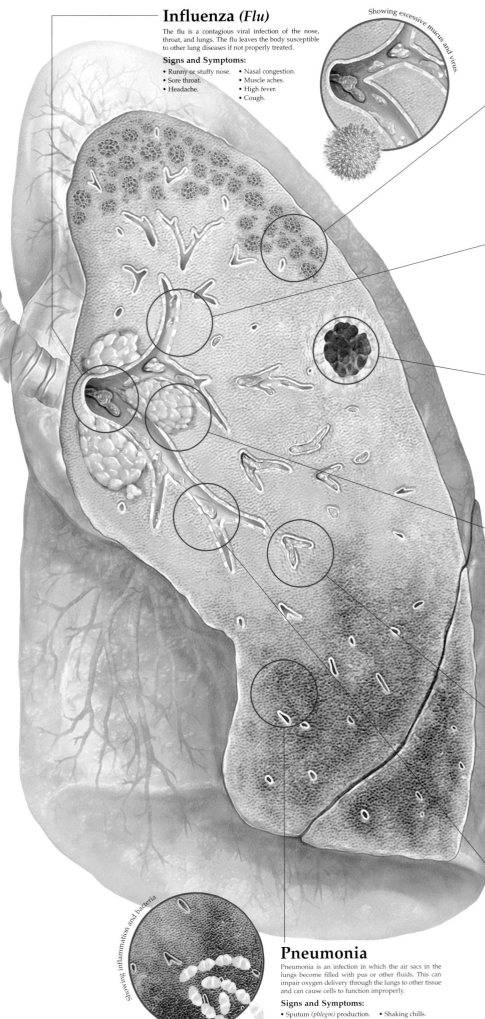

74

Influenza (Flu)

The flu is a contagious viral infection of the nose, throat, and lungs. The flu leaves the body susceptible to other lung diseases if not properly treated.

Signs and Symptoms:

- Runny or stuffy nose.
- Sore throat.
- Headache.
- Nasal congestion.
- Muscle aches.
- High fever.
- Cough.

Showing excessive mucus and virus.

Chronic Obstructive Pulmonary Disease (COPD)

COPD is a disease in which the lung is damaged, making it hard to breathe. It is mainly associated with *chronic bronchitis* and *emphysema*.

Emphysema

Emphysema is a disease that affects the airspaces and tiny blood vessels *(capillaries)* of the lung. The lung tissue loses its recoil ability and the air sacs become enlarged.

Signs and symptoms:

- Prolonged expiration *(breathing out)*.
- Barrel chest *(chest deformity)*.
- Wheezing.
- Dyspnea *(shortness of breath)* with exertion, and later on, even at rest.
- Cough.

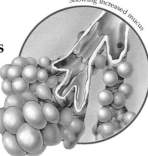

Showing enlarged air sacs

Chronic Bronchitis

Chronic bronchitis is caused by inflammation of the bronchial tube lining. The inflammation leads to increased mucus production and narrowed or blocked airways.

Signs and Symptoms:

- Frequent clearing of the throat.
- Shortness of breath.
- Chronic cough.
- Increased mucus.

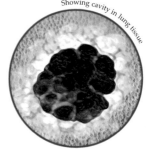

Showing increased mucus

Tuberculosis (TB)

Tuberculosis is an infection caused by the organism *Mycobacterium tuberculosis*. TB is characterized by pulmonary infiltrates *(fluid in the lungs)*, formation of granulomas *(nodular inflammatory injuries)*, fibrosis *(scar tissue)*, and cavitation *(formation of a hollow space in the lung tissue)*.

Signs and Symptoms:

TB is usually without any symptoms but may produce:

- Low-grade fever.
- Loss of appetite.
- Weakness.
- Night sweats.
- Weight-loss.
- Fatigue.

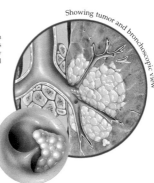

Showing cavity in lung tissue

Lung Cancer

Cancer is a disease in which uncontrolled growth of abnormal cells *(tumor)* crowds out healthy cells and destroys healthy tissue. Lung cancer may develop in the wall of epithelium of the bronchial airway or in the lung tissue itself.

Signs and Symptoms:

- Swelling of the face and neck.
- Unexplained weight loss.
- Swelling of glands in head, neck, or armpits.
- Recurring pneumonia or bronchitis.
- Shortness of breath and wheezing.
- Coughing up blood.
- Persistent cough.
- Loss of appetite.
- Fatigue.
- Chest pain.

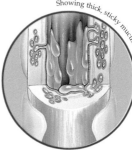

Showing tumor and bronchoscopic view

Cystic Fibrosis

In cystic fibrosis, a defective gene causes the body to produce an abnormally thick, sticky mucus that clogs the lungs and leads to life-threatening lung infections. These thick secretions also obstruct and may destroy the pancreas, preventing digestive enzymes from reaching the intestines to help with break down and absorption of food.

Signs and Symptoms:

- Persistent cough and mucus production.
- Wheezing and shortness of breath.
- Greasy, bulky stools.
- Salty-tasting skin.
- Poor weight gain.
- Recurrent sinus infections.

Showing thick, sticky mucus

Asthma

Asthma is a disease in which the bronchial airways of the lungs become narrow. An asthma episode is the body's reaction to an irritating substance or allergen that has been inhaled. During an asthma episode, the walls of the airways in the lungs become narrowed, thick, and swollen with sticky mucus, making breathing difficult.

Signs and Symptoms:

- Tightness in the neck and/or chest area.
- Wheezing or coughing, especially at night or after exercise.
- Difficulty breathing.
- Symptoms may worsen during an upper respiratory or sinus infection.

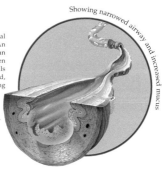

Showing narrowed airway and increased mucus

Pneumonia

Pneumonia is an infection in which the air sacs in the lungs become filled with pus or other fluids. This can impair oxygen delivery through the lungs to other tissue and can cause cells to function improperly.

Signs and Symptoms:

- Sputum *(phlegm)* production.
- Chest pain on inspiration *(breathing in)*.
- Shaking chills.
- Cough.
- Fever.

Showing inflammation and bacteria

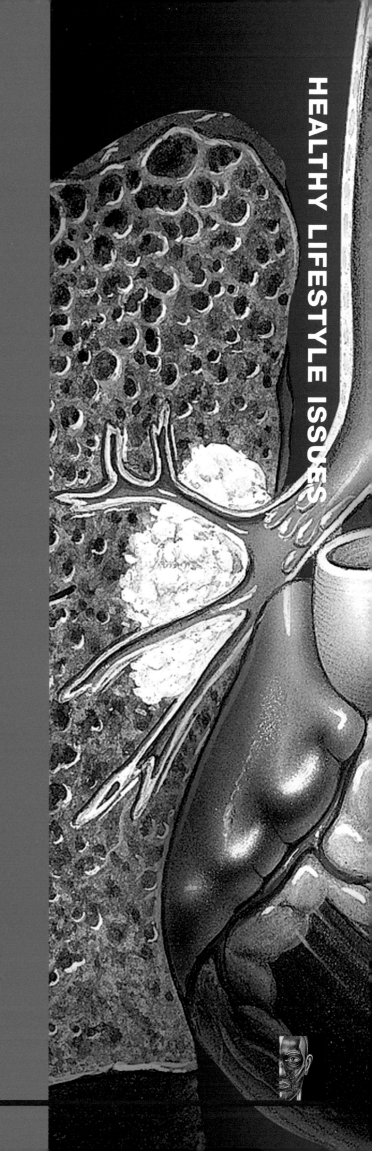

Understanding Menopause

76

Menopause is defined as the date after 12 consistent months without periods. It occurs when the production of the hormones estrogen and progesterone significantly declines. The average age at which menopause occurs in the United States is 52. Menopause is a natural aging process. However, it can also occur due to premature ovarian failure (decreased ovarian hormone production in women under age 40) or surgical removal of the ovaries. Menopause is the start of a menstrual-free lifestyle and no need for birth control.

Perimenopause is the transition into menopause. It can begin as early as a few months to several years prior to menopause and ends with menopause. During this stage, women experience menstrual irregularities (changes in cycle lengths or missed periods) and symptoms of menopause.

What are the Changes I Might Expect?

While some women may only experience the irregularity and eventual ending of menstrual periods, other women may experience a variety of physical and mental/emotional changes.

The most common signs and symptoms of menopause are no periods for 12 months, hot flashes/night sweats, sleep difficulties, and vaginal dryness.

Some changes you may experience:

Hair Growth
- Thinning of scalp hair.
- Darkening/thickening of body hair, such as facial hair.

Breasts and Body changes
- Less firm breasts.
- Weight Gain.

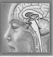

Emotional & Mental Symptoms
- Mood changes/disturbances.
- Irritability.
- Decreased sex drive.
- Lack of concentration/Forgetfulness.
- Depression.
- Nervousness.

Urinary System
- Increased risk of urinary infections.
- Urinary incontinence.

Heart & Circulatory System
- Increased risk of heart disease, high blood pressure, and high cholesterol.

Reproductive System
- Amenorrhea (no more periods).
- Painful intercourse caused by vaginal thinning and dryness.
- Increased risk of vaginal infections.
- Decreased size of fibroids (noncancerous tumors).
- Decreased symptoms of endometriosis (uterus lining grows outside of the uterus) in women who had it prior to menopause.

Skin
- Hot flashes – redness and/or sweating on the face, neck, and chest.
- Sleep disturbances and night sweats (hot flashes occurring at night).
- Thinning of skin, loss of elasticity.
- Sensitivity to sun exposure.

Bone
- Increased risk of osteoporosis (loss of bone mass).

Medications

Other medications for specific symptoms are available; these include medicines for hot flashes, urinary incontinence, and maintenance of bone strength.

Hormone Therapy (HT)

Taking hormone therapy may be a complicated decision for many women; there may be both potential risks and significant benefits to HT. It is important to explore individual risks and benefits with your health care provider before starting HT.

Benefits of Hormone Therapy include:
- Decreased hot flashes
- Decreased vaginal dryness and irritation
- Slowed bone loss and decreased risk of fractures
- Improved sleep/decreased mood swings
- Decreased risk of colorectal cancer (with estrogen plus progestin therapy)

Risks of Hormone Therapy include:
- Blood clots
- Heart attack
- Stroke
- Breast cancer
- Gall bladder disease
- Endometrial cancer (with estrogen alone)

Complementary and Alternative Medicine (CAM)

Talk to your health care provider before starting CAM; some may be beneficial and safe (black cohosh), while others may be ineffective and even dangerous (ginseng, red clover, vitamin E). Current studies do not provide conclusive evidence and more research is being conducted to determined its safety and effectiveness.

Staying Healthy After Menopause

Women should take advantage of preventive options such as:
- Avoid the triggers that can cause hot flashes including:
  - Hot environments
  - Hot or spicy foods
  - Alcohol
  - Caffeine
  - Stress
- Don't smoke.
- Use a water-based vaginal lubricant or moisturizer. Stay sexually active.
- Exercise regularly. Include weight-bearing exercise (such as walking, jogging, or dancing) at least 3 days a week; this may slow down bone loss and improve overall health.
- Get adequate sleep – avoid exercise and alcohol before sleeping.
- Eat a healthy diet that is high in fiber and calcium and low in fat and cholesterol.

In addition to eating right, exercising, getting enough sleep, and avoiding toxins like tobacco and excessive alcohol, it is important to continue regular visits to your health care provider for the following exams and tests:

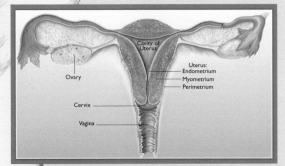

Cavity of Uterus

Ovary

Uterus:
- Endometrium
- Myometrium
- Perimetrium

Cervix

Vagina

The Role of Hormones

The changes experienced during menopause are the body's reaction to the decrease in estrogen and progesterone (hormones produced by the ovaries).

Estrogen
- Declining estrogen production causes inconsistent ovulation and irregular periods.
- Decreased estrogen is also associated with increased risk of heart disease and bone loss.

Progesterone
- Declining progesterone levels may lead to irregular periods and "spotting".

Exam	Frequency
Pelvic exam and Pap smear	Every 2-3 years after 3 consecutive negative annual tests
Breasts exam	Self breast exams once a month and at annual visits
Mammogram	Once every 1-2 years for women age 40–49; every year for women age 50+
Blood work to check thyroid function (TSH test)	Every 5 years
Blood work to check lipid profile (cholesterol & triglyceride levels)	Every 5 years
Fasting glucose (blood sugar) test	Every 3 years
Blood pressure check	At every checkup/exam (at least annually)
Fecal Occult Blood Test (FOBT) – to check for hidden blood in the stool	Annually (may vary based on an individual's risk factors)
Colonoscopy	Every 5 years (may vary based on an individual's risk factors)
Bone scan, such as a DEXA (Dual Energy X-ray absorptiometry scan)	Every 2 years (may vary based on an individual's risk factors)
Skin cancer check	Self skin checks and with annual physical exams (may vary based on an individual's risk factors)

77

Dangers of Alcohol

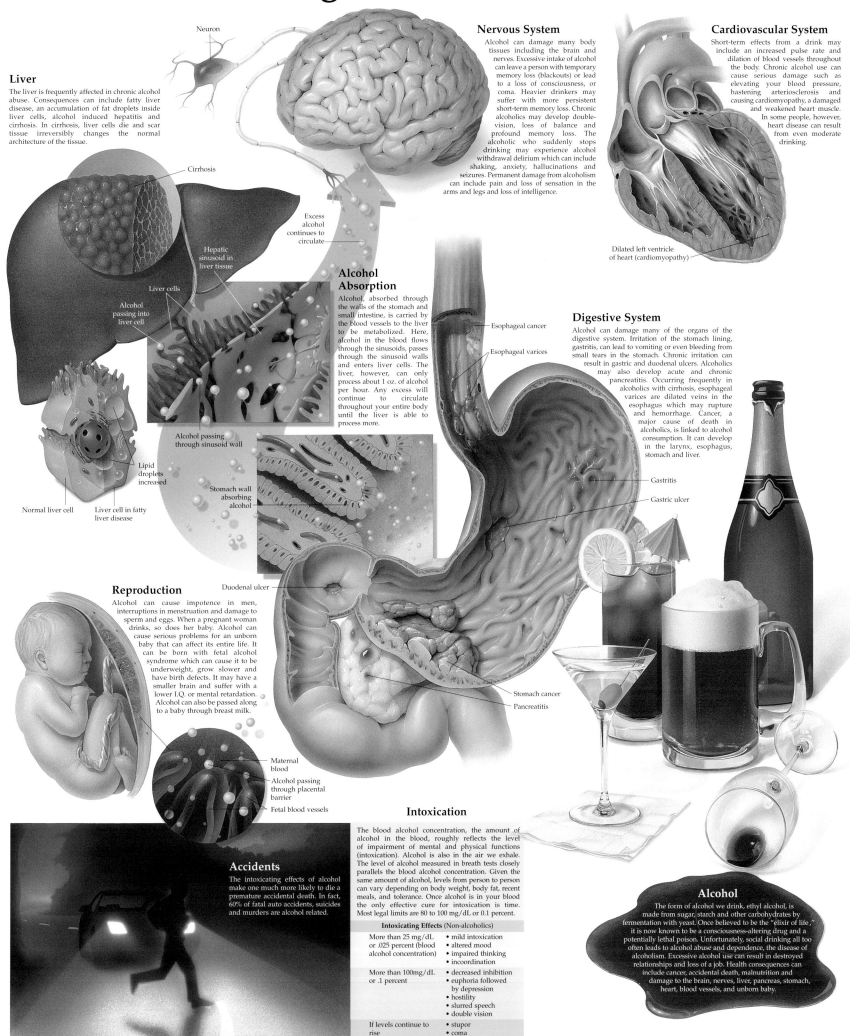

Liver

The liver is frequently affected in chronic alcohol abuse. Consequences can include fatty liver disease, an accumulation of fat droplets inside liver cells, alcohol induced hepatitis and cirrhosis. In cirrhosis, liver cells die and scar tissue irreversibly changes the normal architecture of the tissue.

Cirrhosis

Hepatic sinusoid in liver tissue

Liver cells

Alcohol passing into liver cell

Alcohol passing through sinusoid wall

Lipid droplets increased

Normal liver cell

Liver cell in fatty liver disease

Nervous System

Alcohol can damage many body tissues including the brain and nerves. Excessive intake of alcohol can leave a person with temporary memory loss (blackouts) or lead to a loss of consciousness, or coma. Heavier drinkers may suffer with more persistent short-term memory loss. Chronic alcoholics may develop double-vision, loss of balance and profound memory loss. The alcoholic who suddenly stops drinking may experience alcohol withdrawal delirium which can include shaking, anxiety, hallucinations and seizures. Permanent damage from alcoholism can include pain and loss of sensation in the arms and legs and loss of intelligence.

Neuron

Cardiovascular System

Short-term effects from a drink may include an increased pulse rate and dilation of blood vessels throughout the body. Chronic alcohol use can cause serious damage such as elevating your blood pressure, hastening arteriosclerosis and causing cardiomyopathy, a damaged and weakened heart muscle. In some people, however, heart disease can result from even moderate drinking.

Dilated left ventricle of heart (cardiomyopathy)

Alcohol Absorption

Alcohol, absorbed through the walls of the stomach and small intestine, is carried by the blood vessels to the liver to be metabolized. Here, alcohol in the blood flows through the sinusoids, passes through the sinusoid walls and enters liver cells. The liver, however, can only process about 1 oz. of alcohol per hour. Any excess will continue to circulate throughout your entire body until the liver is able to process more.

Excess alcohol continues to circulate

Esophageal cancer

Esophageal varices

Stomach wall absorbing alcohol

Digestive System

Alcohol can damage many of the organs of the digestive system. Irritation of the stomach lining, gastritis, can lead to vomiting or even bleeding from small tears in the stomach. Chronic irritation can result in gastric and duodenal ulcers. Alcoholics may also develop acute and chronic pancreatitis. Occurring frequently in alcoholics with cirrhosis, esophageal varices are dilated veins in the esophagus which may rupture and hemorrhage. Cancer, a major cause of death in alcoholics, is linked to alcohol consumption. It can develop in the larynx, esophagus, stomach and liver.

Gastritis

Gastric ulcer

Reproduction

Alcohol can cause impotence in men, interruptions in menstruation and damage to sperm and eggs. When a pregnant woman drinks, so does her baby. Alcohol can cause serious problems for an unborn baby that can affect its entire life. It can be born with fetal alcohol syndrome which can cause it to be underweight, grow slower and have birth defects. It may have a smaller brain and suffer with a lower I.Q. or mental retardation. Alcohol can also be passed along to a baby through breast milk.

Duodenal ulcer

Maternal blood

Alcohol passing through placental barrier

Fetal blood vessels

Stomach cancer

Pancreatitis

Intoxication

The blood alcohol concentration, the amount of alcohol in the blood, roughly reflects the level of impairment of mental and physical functions (intoxication). Alcohol is also in the air we exhale. The level of alcohol measured in breath tests closely parallels the blood alcohol concentration. Given the same amount of alcohol, levels from person to person can vary depending on body weight, body fat, recent meals, and tolerance. Once alcohol is in your blood the only effective cure for intoxication is time. Most legal limits are 80 to 100 mg/dL or 0.1 percent.

Accidents

The intoxicating effects of alcohol make one much more likely to die a premature accidental death. In fact, 60% of fatal auto accidents, suicides and murders are alcohol related.

Intoxicating Effects (Non-alcoholics)

More than 25 mg/dL or .025 percent (blood alcohol concentration)	• mild intoxication • altered mood • impaired thinking • incoordination
More than 100mg/dL or .1 percent	• decreased inhibition • euphoria followed by depression • hostility • slurred speech • double vision
If levels continue to rise	• stupor • coma

Alcohol

The form of alcohol we drink, ethyl alcohol, is made from sugar, starch and other carbohydrates by fermentation with yeast. Once believed to be the "elixir of life," it is now known to be a consciousness-altering drug and a potentially lethal poison. Unfortunately, social drinking all too often leads to alcohol abuse and dependence, the disease of alcoholism. Excessive alcohol use can result in destroyed relationships and loss of a job. Health consequences can include cancer, accidental death, malnutrition and damage to the brain, nerves, liver, pancreas, stomach, heart, blood vessels, and unborn baby.

Dangers of Smoking

78

Tobacco smoke is a highly dangerous substance that contains more than 200 known poisons. Every time a smoker lights up, he or she is being injured to some degree by inhaling these poisons. A two-pack-a-day smoker shortens his or her life expectancy by eight years, and even light smokers shorten their life expectancy by four years. To date, lung cancer is the leading cause of death in men, yet incidence is increasing among women often resulting in death at an earlier age than men.

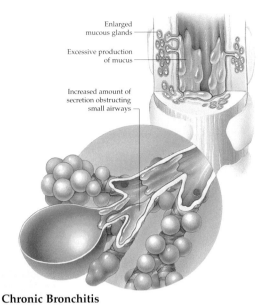

Enlarged mucous glands

Excessive production of mucus

Increased amount of secretion obstructing small airways

Chronic Bronchitis

A persistent cough is the major symptom of chronic bronchitis. In the large airways, the size and number of mucus-secreting glands are increased. In the small airways, there are increased secretions, impaired handling of secretions, and inflammation that can impair or obstruct air flow.

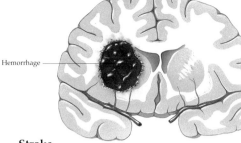

Hemorrhage

Stroke

Smoking is a major cause of arteriosclerosis, or hardening of the arteries. In turn, arteriosclerosis is a chief cause of stroke. Strokes occur when one of the arteries of the brain ruptures, forms a blood clot, or bleeds into the brain. Once brain tissue is destroyed it cannot be repaired.

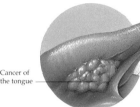

Brain

Tongue

Mouth and Throat Cancer

Cancer-causing chemicals from tobacco products increase the risk of cancer of the lip, cheek, tongue, and larynx (voice box). The removal of these cancers can be disfiguring and can result in loss of the larynx.

Cancer of the tongue

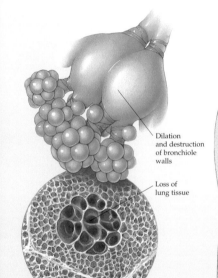

Dilation and destruction of bronchiole walls

Loss of lung tissue

Emphysema

With emphysema, the lungs irreversibly lose their ability to take up oxygen, causing great breathing difficulty. Lung tissue loses its elasticity, air sacs tear, and stale air becomes trapped, eventually causing death from lack of oxygen.

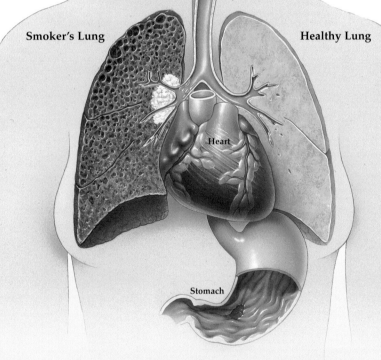

Smoker's Lung

Healthy Lung

Heart

Stomach

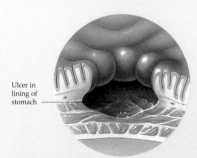

Plaque in coronary artery wall

Heart Disease

Arteriosclerosis is responsible for most heart attacks. Plaque, deposits of cholesterol, collecting in the coronary arteries narrows the vessels until eventually the oxygen supply to the heart is stopped. Smoking accelerates this process.

Ulcer in lining of stomach

Gastric Ulcer

Smoking increases the production of gastric juices, raising the acidity level and eroding the lining of the stomach. Painful ulcers result from these eroded areas and increase the risk for hemorrhage and perforation of the stomach lining.

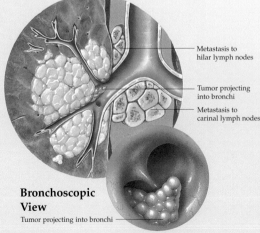

Metastasis to hilar lymph nodes

Tumor projecting into bronchi

Metastasis to carinal lymph nodes

Bronchoscopic View

Tumor projecting into bronchi

Lung Cancer

Tobacco smoke is the most common cause of lung cancer. One in ten heavy smokers will get lung cancer, and in most cases it will be fatal. It is the leading cause of death by cancer because it is difficult to detect, and it is likely to spread early to the liver, brain, and bones.

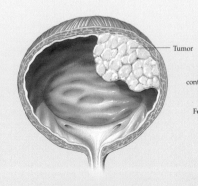

Tumor

Bladder Cancer

Chemicals from tobacco are absorbed into the bloodstream and leave the body through the urine. These cancer-causing chemicals are always in contact with the bladder, increasing the risk for bladder cancer.

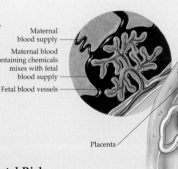

Maternal blood supply

Maternal blood containing chemicals mixes with fetal blood supply

Fetal blood vessels

Placenta

Fetal Risk

Carbon monoxide in smoke reduces the oxygen level in the fetus' (unborn child's) blood, while nicotine restricts the blood flow from the mother to the fetus. Smoking is thought to retard the growth of the fetus, resulting in low birth weight. Smoking also increases the risk of premature birth and infant death.

79

BMI & Waist Circumference

Body Mass Index (BMI)

The BMI (Body Mass Index) is a way to interpret the risk of weight for your height. The higher the BMI, the higher the risk.

English Formula

$$BMI = \frac{weight\ in\ pounds}{(height\ in\ inches) \times (height\ in\ inches)} \times 703$$

Metric Formula

$$BMI = \frac{weight\ in\ kilograms}{(height\ in\ meters) \times (height\ in\ meters)}$$

BMI does have some limitations:

- It may overestimate body fat in athletes or people with muscular build.
- It may underestimate body fat in older person and others who have lost muscle mass.
- There may be differences in what constitutes healthy and unhealthy BMIs among different ethnic groups, such as people of Asian descent.

Waist Circumference

The waist circumference measurement is useful in assessing risk for adults who are normal or overweight according to the BMI table. It is a good indicator of abdominal fat.

People with high-risk waist lines are at higher risk for developing other diseases such as diabetes, hypertension (high blood pressure), dyslipidemia (which are abnormal blood fats such as high LDL cholesterol, high triglycerides and/or low HDL cholesterol), and cardiovascular disease.

High-Risk Waist Line

For Men: Over 40 inches (102 cm)
For Women: Over 35 inches (88 cm)

If a patient has a normal or overweight BMI and has a high-risk waist line, they are considered one (1) risk category above that defined by their BMI. Please note that there may be differences in what constitutes a higher risk waist line among different ethnic groups.

How to measure: The measurement for waist circumference is at the ILIAC CREST.

Classification	BMI
Underweight	Below 18.5
Normal	18.5 – 24.9
Overweight	25.0 – 29.9
Obese Class I	30.0- 34.9
Obese Class II	35.0 – 39.9
Obese Class III (Extreme Obesity)	40.0+

Body Mass Index (BMI) Table

To determine your BMI, look down the left column to find your height and then look across that row and find the weight that is nearest your own. Now look to the top of the column to find the number that is your BMI.

	Normal						Overweight					Obese										Extreme Obesity															
BMI	19	20	21	22	23	24	25	26	27	28	29	30	31	32	33	34	35	36	37	38	39	40	41	42	43	44	45	46	47	48	49	50	51	52	53	54
Height (feet & inches)												Body Weight (pounds)																								
4'10" (58")	91	96	100	105	110	115	119	124	129	134	138	143	148	153	158	162	167	172	177	181	186	191	196	201	205	210	215	220	224	229	234	239	244	248	253	258
4'11" (59")	94	99	104	109	114	119	124	128	133	138	143	148	153	158	163	168	173	178	183	188	193	198	203	208	212	217	222	227	232	237	242	247	252	257	262	267
5'0" (60")	97	102	107	112	118	123	128	133	138	143	148	153	158	163	168	174	179	184	189	194	199	204	209	215	220	225	230	235	240	245	250	255	261	266	271	276
5'1" (61")	100	106	111	116	122	127	132	137	143	148	153	158	164	169	174	180	185	190	195	201	206	211	217	222	227	232	238	243	248	254	259	264	269	275	280	285
5'2" (62")	104	109	115	120	126	131	136	142	147	153	158	164	169	175	180	186	191	196	202	207	213	218	224	229	235	240	246	251	256	262	267	273	278	284	289	295
5'3" (63")	107	113	118	124	130	135	141	146	152	158	163	169	175	180	186	191	197	203	208	214	220	225	231	237	242	248	254	259	265	270	278	282	287	293	299	304
5'4" (64")	110	116	122	128	134	140	145	151	157	163	169	174	180	186	192	197	204	209	215	221	227	232	238	244	250	256	262	267	273	279	285	291	296	302	308	314
5'5" (65")	114	120	126	132	138	144	150	156	162	168	174	180	186	192	198	204	210	216	222	228	234	240	246	252	258	264	270	276	282	288	294	300	306	312	318	324
5'6" (66")	118	124	130	136	142	148	155	161	167	173	179	186	192	198	204	210	216	223	229	235	241	247	253	260	266	272	278	284	291	297	303	309	315	322	328	334
5'7" (67")	121	127	134	140	146	153	159	166	172	178	185	191	198	204	211	217	223	230	236	242	249	255	261	268	274	280	287	293	299	306	312	319	325	331	338	344
5'8" (68")	125	131	138	144	151	158	164	171	177	184	190	197	203	210	216	223	230	236	243	249	256	262	269	276	282	289	295	302	308	315	322	328	335	341	348	354
5'9" (69")	128	135	142	149	155	162	169	176	182	189	196	203	209	216	223	230	236	243	250	257	263	270	277	284	291	297	304	311	318	324	331	338	345	351	358	365
5'10" (70")	132	139	146	153	160	167	174	181	188	195	202	209	216	222	229	236	243	250	257	264	271	278	285	292	299	306	313	320	327	334	341	348	355	362	369	376
5'11" (71")	136	143	150	157	165	172	179	186	193	200	208	215	222	229	236	243	250	257	265	272	279	286	293	301	308	315	322	329	338	343	351	358	365	372	379	386
6'0" (72")	140	147	154	162	169	177	184	191	199	206	213	221	228	235	242	250	258	265	272	279	287	294	302	309	316	324	331	338	346	353	361	368	375	383	390	397
6'1" (73")	144	151	159	166	174	182	189	197	204	212	219	227	235	242	250	257	265	272	280	288	295	302	310	318	325	333	340	348	355	363	371	378	386	393	401	408
6'2" (74")	148	155	163	171	179	186	194	202	210	218	225	233	241	249	256	264	272	280	287	295	303	311	319	326	334	342	350	358	365	373	381	389	396	404	412	420
6'3" (75")	152	160	168	176	184	192	200	208	216	224	232	240	248	256	264	272	279	287	295	303	311	319	327	335	343	351	359	367	375	383	391	399	407	415	423	431
6'4" (76")	156	164	172	180	189	197	205	213	221	230	238	246	254	263	271	279	287	295	304	312	320	328	336	344	353	361	369	377	385	394	402	410	418	426	435	443

Source: National Heart, Lung, and Blood Institute.

©2008 Wolters Kluwer Health | Lippincott Williams & Wilkins | Published by Anatomical Chart Company, Skokie, IL

80

Daily Goal:
Carbohydrates should contribute 55-60% of total calories, mostly from complex carbohydrates (whole grain breads and cereals, fruits and vegetables).

Daily Goal:
Protein intake should be 15-20% of total calories.

Daily Goal:
Fiber intake should be about 25-30g per day.

Daily Goal:
Dietary fat should contribute 25-35% of total caloric intake, with no more than 10% of these calories from saturated fat.

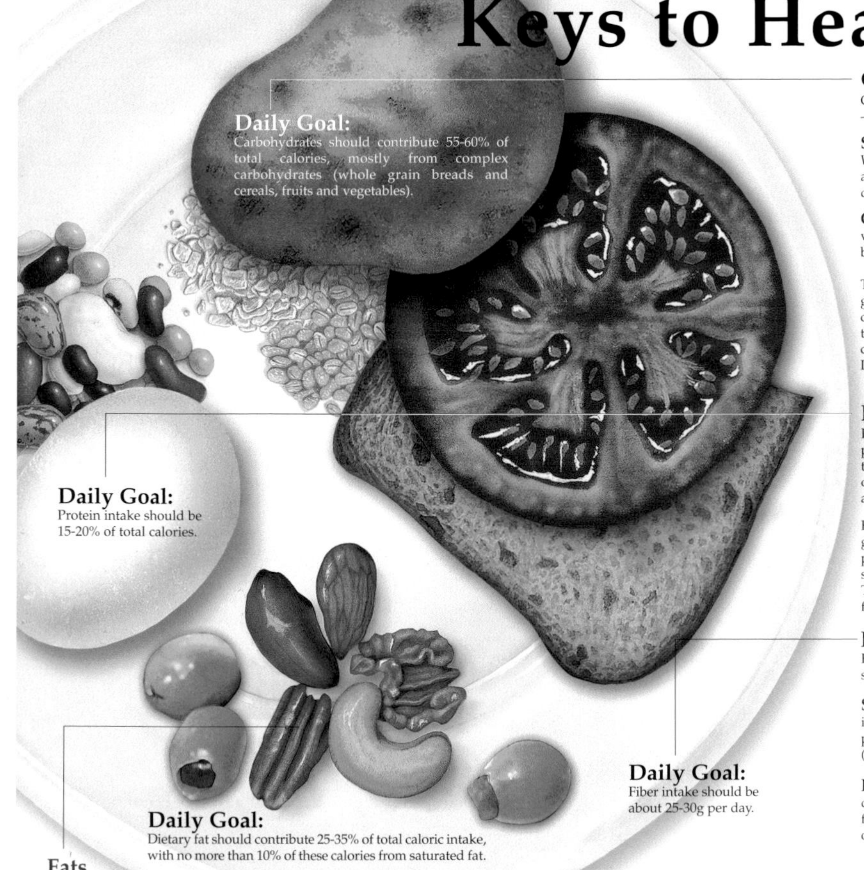

Carbohydrates

Carbohydrates are the primary energy source that fuels the body. There are two categories of carbohydrates – simple and complex.

Simple carbohydrates are sugars that provide the body with energy (calories) but little nutrition. White and brown sugar, honey, sugar naturally found in fruit, and high fructose corn syrup (widely used as a sweetener) are some examples. Simple sugars should be limited because they increase the risk of developing dental problems, type 2 diabetes, and obesity.

Complex carbohydrates are the body's primary source of energy. They are also packed with a rich variety of vitamins, minerals, fiber, and phytochemicals (plant nutrients). Fruits; vegetables; whole grain breads, cereals, and pasta; dried beans; nuts; and seeds are excellent examples of complex carbohydrates.

The **Glycemic Index** (GI) describes the rate of carbohydrate digestion. GI measures how quickly 100 grams of a carbohydrate-rich food is processed by the body. Highly processed foods containing simple carbohydrates, such as white bread, sweets, and some snack foods have a high GI and the body digests them rapidly, causing spikes in blood sugar levels. On the other hand, whole grain, complex carbohydrates such as dried beans, lentils, and oatmeal have a low GI and stabilize blood glucose levels. Low GI foods are thought to decrease the risk of type 2 diabetes, obesity, and cardiovascular disease.

Protein

Protein is the basic structural material of all cells. In the body, biologically active proteins include enzymes, hormones, and neurotransmitters. Twenty **amino acids**, the building blocks of dietary protein, are found in both plant and animal foods. Nine of these amino acids are considered "essential" because they cannot be made in the body and must be acquired from food.

Eating a combination of heart-healthy plant protein sources such as nuts, legumes, and whole grains can meet the body's requirement for essential amino acids. Meat, poultry and dairy products are also complete protein sources, but many animal protein foods are rich in saturated fat and dietary cholesterol, which can negatively impact heart health. These substances may also tax the kidneys by promoting kidney stones or form and increasing urinary calcium losses, a risk factor for osteoporosis.

Fiber

Fiber is a key health benefit of a diet rich in whole grains, fruits, vegetables, legumes, nuts and seeds. A high fiber diet is associated with reduced risk of cancer, heart disease, type 2 diabetes, and obesity.

Soluble fiber helps lower blood cholesterol and glucose (sugar) levels. Fiber is categorized by its solubility ability to dissolve in water. Food sources rich in soluble fiber include oatmeal, barley, pectin-rich fruit (apples, pears, plums, strawberries), dried beans, and some vegetables (artichokes, peas, carrots, and brussels sprouts).

Insoluble fiber is a component of plant foods that cannot be broken down by the digestive system. Whole grain cereal, bread, rice, and pasta are the best sources of insoluble fiber in the American diet. These foods may help in weight loss because it creates a feeling of fullness for long periods of time, which may make overeating less likely.

Fats

In food, fat is the greatest dietary energy source. It also plays an important role in the digestion, absorption, and transport of fat-soluble nutrients – vitamins A, D, E, and K.

Some fat tissue is essential because it provides structural functions like supporting cell walls, padding vital organs, and insulating the body. However, overconsumption of calories from fat or other energy sources is stored as excess body fat, which is not healthy.

Cholesterol is a waxlike substance that is transported throughout the body in the form of lipoprotein (fat bound with protein). LDL and HDL, the two primary lipoproteins, have opposite effects on heart health.

LDL (low-density lipoprotein) is considered "bad" because it deposits cholesterol into coronary arteries. Over time, this plaque buildup narrows the opening of these arteries, which significantly increases the risk of a heart attack.

HDL (high-density lipoprotein) is "good" because it carries cholesterol back to the liver for reprocessing, which eventually eliminates it from the body. High blood levels of HDL help reduce the risk of heart disease.

Fats in food can have either positive or negative effects on blood cholesterol levels. Unsaturated fats have the most favorable impact on heart health.

"Good" Fats

Monounsaturated fat: Lowers LDL, raises HDL, decreases risk of heart disease. Sources: Peanuts, nuts, olives, olive oil, canola oil, avocados

Polyunsaturated fat: Lowers LDL, may lower HDL, may decrease risk of heart disease. Sources: Corn, soybean, safflower, and cottonseed oils.

Omega-3 polyunsaturated fat: Lowers LDL and triglycerides, reduces the risk of blood clotting, lowers blood pressure. Sources: Salmon, mackerel, flaxseed, canola oil, walnuts.

"Bad" Fats

Saturated fat: Raises LDL, increases risk of heart disease. Sources: Red meat, sausage, processed meats, cheese, whole milk, cream, ice cream, baked goods, chocolate candy.

Trans fat: Raises LDL, lowers HDL, increases risk of heart disease. Sources: Fried chicken, french fries, doughnuts, and other deep-fried food; movie popcorn; partially hydrogenated stick margarine; shortenings; some commercial baked goods.

How to Use the Food Pyramid

MyPyramid, an updated version of the Food Guide Pyramid, was developed to be consistent with USDA dietary guidelines. This graphical representation of a nutritious diet guides consumers on how to choose the right types and amounts of foods to eat as part of a healthy lifestyle.

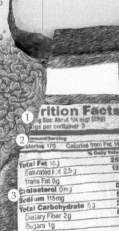

MyPyramid.gov
STEPS TO A HEALTHIER YOU

The color-coded vertical slices of the pyramid correspond with each of the six food groups. Fruits, vegetables, and grains, the wider sections of the pyramid, are the recommended staples of a balanced diet.

Variety and proportionality of all food groups are also emphasized in MyPyramid (available at www.mypyramid.gov). A personalized feature of this pyramid is an online interactive tool that calculates an adult's suggested daily calorie needs (based on height, weight, and activity level) and recommends portions to eat from each food group. Additionally, the climbing figure across the side of the pyramid underscores the importance of daily physical activity for weight control.

How to Read a Nutrition Label

(1) **Serving Size:** Compare the serving size listed on the label with your own portion and then multiply each nutrient accordingly. For example, if a serving of cereal is 1 cup and you've poured yourself 2 cups, you must double all the nutrient values on the label (e.g., 2 g of fat/serving becomes 4 g).

Consumers should be aware that the amount of food contained in what looks like a single-serving package, like a small bag of chips, may be more than one serving, and thus may not be an appropriate portion size.

(2) **Calories:** More than half of Americans are overweight or obese. Hence, consumers are advised to watch their calorie intake. According to the Food and Drug Administration, 40 calories per serving is low, 100 calories is moderate, and 400 calories or more is high.

(3)(4) **Nutrients:** Eating too much saturated and trans fat, dietary cholesterol, and sodium is linked to heart disease, some cancers, and obesity. These nutrients are typically over-consumed by many Americans and therefore should be limited as much as possible (3).

Many American adults do not get their daily requirement of fiber, vitamins A and C, calcium, and iron. Lacking these nutrients can contribute to diseases such as certain cancers, osteoporosis, and anemia. Consumers should make sure their intake of these vitamins and minerals is adequate (4).

(5) **Footnote:** The Daily Values (DV) that were determined by public health and nutrition experts are listed in the footnote section of the nutrition label. DV, or recommended intakes for certain nutrients, are based on a 2000-calorie diet. Consumers should be aware of the following statement, which precedes the DV information: "Percent Daily Values are based on a 2,000 calorie diet. Your Daily Values may be higher or lower depending on your calorie needs."

(6) **% Daily Value:** The percent DV is shown in the right-hand column of the nutrition label. Keep in mind that the DV is based on the serving amount. If a larger portion is consumed, the percent DV needs to be multiplied accordingly. Consumers can use the following guidelines when interpreting the DV percentages: 5% DV or less is low; 20% DV or more is high. *Note: Trans fat does not have a DV because this type of fat should be avoided as much as possible.*

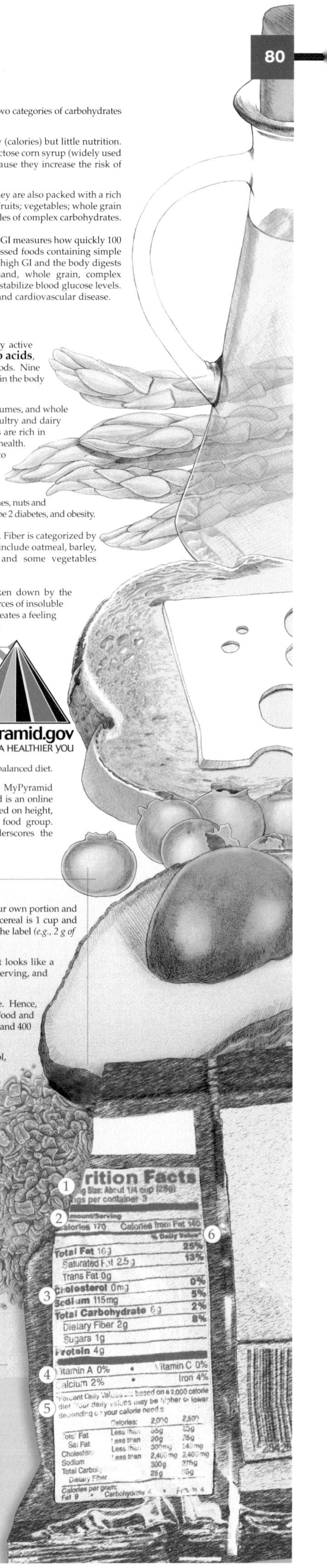

Vitamins

There are many vitamins and minerals that make up a healthy, nutritionally balanced diet. These elements are needed to convert food to energy, create amino and fatty acids, generate tissue growth, and drive many other internal processes. Generally, a varied diet including whole grain foods, lean meat, vegetables, legumes, fruits, and nuts is an excellent source of essential vitamins and minerals.

Note: Some nutrient are particularly important to certain age groups (as demonstrated below), but it is important to balance these nutrients at all stages of life. Check with your doctor for your specific needs.

	RDA	Benefits	Sources	Children (2yrs. +)	Adolescents	Women*	All Adults	Seniors
Vitamin A	700-900 mcg	• Night vision • Growth and tissue healing • Maintaining healthy skin	Cheese; eggs; chicken; salmon; yellow, orange, and leafy dark green vegetables					
Vitamin B₁₂	1-2.4 mcg	• DNA metabolism • Red blood cell formation • Central nervous system maintenance	Milk, eggs, yogurt, fish, shellfish, red meat, fortified cereals					
Vitamin C	45-90 mg	• Controls infections • Powerful antioxidant • Helps make collagen	Citrus fruit, broccoli, berries, green and red peppers, spinach, fortified cereals					
Vitamin D	5-10 mcg	Maintenance of bones and teeth	Fortified milk and cereal, egg yolks, butter, salmon, mild exposure to sunlight 30 minutes/week					
Vitamin E	15 mg	• Protects muscle and red blood cells • Antioxidant benefits • Helps the body use vitamins A & K	Nuts, seeds, vegetable oils, whole grains, leafy greens					
Calcium	1000 mg	Maintenance of bones and teeth	Milk, yogurt, cheese, ice cream, salmon, broccoli, kale, collard greens, mustard greens, spinach					
Fiber	20-35 g	• Prevents constipation • Stabilizes blood sugar levels • May lower blood cholesterol	Vegetables, bran, whole grains, whole fruits, seeds, oatmeal,barley, popcorn					
Folic Acid	400 mcg	• Protects against neurological birth defects • Improves heart health	Asparagus, broccoli, avocados, beans, soybeans, lentils, oranges, peas, turkey, bok choy, spinach					
Iron	8-18 mg	Formation of hemoglobin which blood cells use to carry oxygen to the body	Beef, chicken, tuna, shrimp, dried beans, nuts, spinach, whole grains, strawberries					
Magnesium	300-400 mg	• Promotes proper nerve function • Helps the body use insulin • Helps the body make bone and teeth	Whole grains, nuts, beans seeds, fish, avocados, leafy green vegetables					
Potassium (vitamin K)	90-120 mg	• Promotes blood clotting • Regulates water balance • Helps maintain blood pressure	Green vegetables, brussels sprouts, yogurt, avocados, bananas, orange juice, potatoes					
Zinc	8-11 mg	• Reduces inflammation • Boosts the immune system • Production of DNA	Meat, poultry, oysters, eggs, milk products, legumes, seeds, nuts					

* of child-bearing age

Portion Guide:

Use these everyday objects to remember the proper serving sizes of common foods.

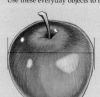

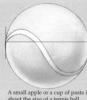

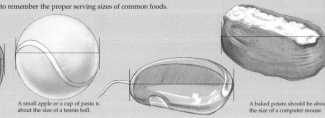

A small apple or a cup of pasta is about the size of a tennis ball.

A baked potato should be about the size of a computer mouse.

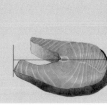

A 3 oz. piece of meat or fish should be about the size of your fist.

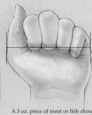

Nutrition Facts
Serving Size: About 1/4 cup (28g)
Servings per container: 3

Amount/Serving
Calories 170   Calories from Fat 146

	% Daily Value*
Total Fat 16g	25%
Saturated Fat 2.5g	13%
Trans Fat 0g	
Cholesterol 0mg	0%
Sodium 115mg	5%
Total Carbohydrate 6g	2%
Dietary Fiber 2g	8%
Sugars 1g	
Protein 4g	

| Vitamin A 0% | Vitamin C 0% |
| Calcium 2% | Iron 4% |

Percent Daily Values are based on a 2,000 calorie diet. Your daily values may be higher or lower depending on your calorie needs:

	Calories:	2,000	2,500
Total Fat	Less than	65g	75g
Sat Fat	Less than	20g	25g
Cholesterol	Less than	300mg	300mg
Sodium	Less than	2,400mg	2,400mg
Total Carb.		300g	375g
Dietary Fiber		25g	35g

Calories per gram:
Fat 9   Carbohydrate 4   Protein 4

81

Maintaining a Healthy Weight

Healthy Diet Plan

If you are concerned about your diet, no particular food plan is magical and no particular food must be either included or avoided. Your diet should consist of foods that you like or can learn to like, that are available to you, and that are within your means. The most effective diet programs for weight loss and maintenance are based on physical activity and reasonable serving sizes, with less frequent consumption of foods high in fat and refined sugars.

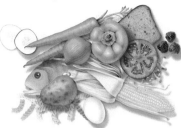

Physiological Hazards That Accompany Low-Carbohydrate Diets

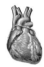

- **Heart Failure**
  Carbohydrates maintain sodium and fluid balance. A carbohydrate deficiency promotes loss of sodium and water, which can adversely affect blood pressure and cardiac function if not corrected.

- **High Blood Cholesterol**
  Low-carbohydrate diets can raise blood cholesterol because in these diets, fruits, vegetables, breads, and cereals are replaced by meat and dairy products, which are rich in fat and protein. High fat and protein intakes, especially from meat and dairy products, raise LDL and total cholesterol.

- **Metabolic Abnormalities**
  When carbohydrate intake is low, ketones are produced from fat to replace carbohydrates as a source of energy for the brain. Since ketones are acids, high levels can make the blood acidic, altering respiration and other metabolic processes that are sensitive to an increase or decrease in acidity.

The Risk in Low-Carbohydrate Diets

Low-carbohydrate diets, especially if undertaken without medical supervision, can be dangerous. Low-carbohydrate diets are designed to cause rapid weight loss by promoting an undesirably high concentration of ketone bodies (a byproduct of fat metabolism). The sales pitch is that you'll never feel hungry and that you'll lose weight faster than you would on any "ordinary diet". Both claims are true but the low-carb diets are true but misleading. Fast weight loss means loss of water and lean tissue, which are rapidly regained when people begin eating their usual diets again. The amount of body fat lost, will be the same as with a conventional low- calorie diet. Fat loss is always equal to the difference between energy consumed in food and energy expended in activity.

Overweight Problems

As the amount of body fat increases, especially around the abdomen, so does the risk of:

- Respiratory disease
- Obstructive sleep apnea
- Complications during surgery
- Gallbladder disease
- Stroke
- Non-insulin-dependent (type 2) diabetes
- Some forms of cancer, especially breast and colon
- Coronary heart disease
- Hypertension

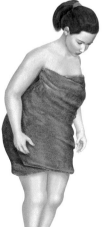

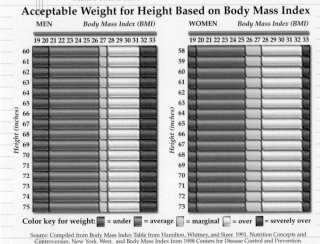

Strategies for Diet Planning:

- Adopt a realistic long-term plan.
- Individualize your diet, include foods that you like, and indulge yourself once in a while.
  - Include foods from all five food groups.
  - Eat foods that contain a lot of nutrients.
  - Stress the Dos and not the Don'ts in your diet and your way of living.
  - Eat on a regular schedule at least 3 times a day. Don't skip meals.

Suggestions and Tips for Physical Activity:

- Walk at least 10-20 minutes daily.
- Take the stairs instead of the elevator.
- Sports (basketball, baseball, tennis...)
- Dance classes
- Aerobics classes
- Incorporate exercise into your normal routine.
- Concentrate on strengthening your muscles as well as your heart and lungs.

What Is Your Body Mass Index?

Your body mass index (**BMI**) is your weight in kilograms divided by the square of your height in meters. It is used to indicate whether or not you are overweight or underweight.

How to Calculate Your Body Mass Index:

1. Convert your weight in pounds (lb) to kilograms (kg) by dividing your weight in pounds by 2.2 kg.
2. Convert your height in inches (in.) to meters (m) by multiplying your height in inches by .0254 m.
3. Take your height in meters and square it by multiplying it by itself.
4. Divide your weight in kilograms by your height in meters squared (your calculated height from step 3).

Example: Mark weighs 150 lb and is 5 ft, 10 in. tall (70 in.).
1. 150 lb ÷ by 2.2 kg = 68.18 kg
2. 70 in. x .0254 m = 1.778 m
3. 1.778 m x 1.778 m = 3.161 m²
4. 68.18 kg ÷ 3.161 m² = 21.56

Mark's BMI is 21.56

Acceptable Weight for Height Based on Body Mass Index

MEN — *Body Mass Index (BMI)*
19 20 21 22 23 24 25 26 27 28 29 30 31 32 33
Height (inches): 60 61 62 63 64 65 66 67 68 69 70 71 72 73 74 75

WOMEN — *Body Mass Index (BMI)*
19 20 21 22 23 24 25 26 27 28 29 30 31 32 33
Height (inches): 58 59 60 61 62 63 64 65 66 67 68 69 70 71 72 73

Color key for weight: ■ = under ■ = average ■ = marginal ■ = over ■ = severely over

Source: Compiled from Body Mass Index Table from Hamilton, Whitney, and Sizer. 1991. Nutrition Concepts and Controversies. New York. West. and Body Mass Index from 1998 Centers for Disease Control and Prevention.

Excess Fat Distribution

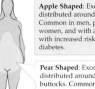
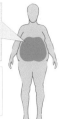

Apple Shaped: Excess fat is distributed around the abdomen. Common in men, postmenopausal women, and with aging. Associated with increased risk of Type 2 diabetes.

Pear Shaped: Excess fat is distributed around the hips and buttocks. Common in women. Associated with increased risk of osteoarthritis.

Understanding Calories

Calories are a standard measurement of heat energy. Technically, 1 calorie is 1 kilocalorie, which is the amount of heat required to raise the temperature of 1 kg. of water by 1°C.

A person's energy needs are determined by the amount of lean tissue or muscle and by the level of activity. A small, elderly, sedentary woman may need only about 1,200 calories to meet her energy needs each day, while a tall, young, physically active man may need as many as 4,000 calories daily.

How to Calculate Your Total Daily Energy (Calorie) Needs

1. Convert your weight from pounds (lb) to kilograms (kg) by dividing your weight in pounds by 2.2 lb/kg.
2. Multiply your weight in kilograms by 30 kcal/kg if you are a man and 25 kcal/kg if you are a woman.

Example
1. 150 lb ÷ by 2.2 lb/kg = 68.18 kg
2. 68.18 kg x 30 kcal/kg = 2,045 kcal

Result: A 150 lb man needs approximately 2,045 kcal (calories) a day to maintain his weight.

Energy Demands of Activities

Activity	Body Weight (lb)				
	110	125	150	175	200
	CALORIES PER MINUTE				
Aerobics	6.8	7.8	9.3	10.9	12.4
Basketball (vigorous)	10.7	12.1	14.6	17.0	19.4
Bicycling					
13 miles per hour	5.0	5.6	6.8	7.9	9.0
Cross-country skiing					
8 miles per hour	11.4	13.0	15.6	18.2	20.8
Golf (carrying clubs)	5.0	5.6	6.8	7.9	9.0
Rowing (vigorous)	10.7	12.1	14.6	17.0	19.4
Running					
5 miles per hour	6.7	7.6	9.2	10.7	12.2
Soccer	10.7	2.1	14.6	17.0	19.4
Studying	1.2	1.4	1.7	1.9	2.2
Swimming					
20 yards per minute	3.5	4.0	4.8	5.6	6.4
Walking (brisk pace)					
3.5 miles per hour	3.9	4.4	5.2	6.1	7.0

Source: Compiled from Hamilton, Whitney, and Sizer. 1991. Nutrition Concepts and Controversies. New York. West.

Underweight Problems

When body weight decreases to 15-20% below desirable weight (BMI < 18.5), the amount of energy being consumed is not sufficient to support the function of vital organs. Lean tissue is being broken down and utilized for energy to make up the deficit. The results are:

- Low body temperature
- Abnormal electrical activity in the brain
- Altered blood lipids
- Dry skin
- Impaired immune response
- Loss of digestive function
- Abnormal hormone levels
- Malnutrition
- Anemia

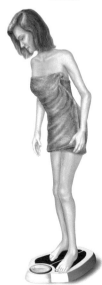

©2008 Wolters Kluwer | Lippincott Williams & Wilkins | Published by Anatomical Chart Company, Skokie, IL

82

Risks of Obesity

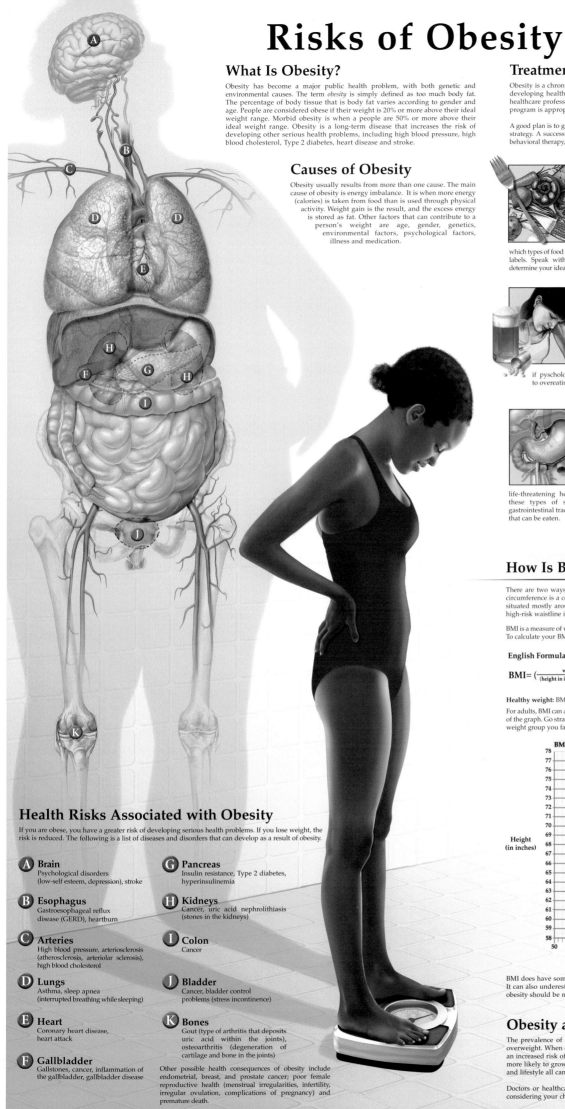

What Is Obesity?

Obesity has become a major public health problem, with both genetic and environmental causes. The term *obesity* is simply defined as too much body fat. The percentage of body tissue that is body fat varies according to gender and age. People are considered obese if their weight is 20% or more above their ideal weight range. Morbid obesity is when a people are 50% or more above their ideal weight range. Obesity is a long-term disease that increases the risk of developing other serious health problems, including high blood pressure, high blood cholesterol, Type 2 diabetes, heart disease and stroke.

Causes of Obesity

Obesity usually results from more than one cause. The main cause of obesity is energy imbalance. It is when more energy (calories) is taken from food than is used through physical activity. Weight gain is the result, and the excess energy is stored as fat. Other factors that can contribute to a person's weight are age, gender, genetics, environmental factors, psychological factors, illness and medication.

Treatment for Adult Obesity

Obesity is a chronic disease and it needs long-term management. The focus usually is to reduce the risk for developing health problems, as well as to lose the excess weight. If you are obese, it is best to consult a healthcare professional to help determine how much weight you should lose and what kind of weight loss program is appropriate.

A good plan is to gradually reduce your weight. Weight loss of one to two pounds per week is a safe and healthy strategy. A successful treatment plan can include one or more of the following options: diet, physical activity, behavioral therapy, counseling, drug therapy, and surgery.

Diet

For weight loss, a low calorie, well-balanced diet that is low in fat is recommended. Dietary therapy involves reducing the number of calories that are eaten and learning how to select portion sizes, which types of food to buy, and how to read nutrition labels. Speak with a healthcare professional to determine your ideal calorie intake.

Physical Activity

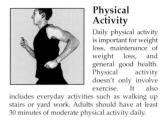

Daily physical activity is important for weight loss, maintenance of weight loss, and general good health. Physical activity doesn't only involve exercise. It also includes everyday activities such as walking up stairs or yard work. Adults should have at least 30 minutes of moderate physical activity daily.

Counseling

Sometimes, social problems (alcohol or drugs) or psychological problems (depression or anxiety) play an important part in weight gain. Individual or group counseling is an important treatment if pyschological or social problems lead to overeating.

Drug Therapy

If prescribed, drug treatment should be used in combination with a healthy diet and physical activity. Patients should have regular visits with their healthcare professional to monitor their progress and any side effects the medication may have.

Surgery

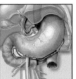

Surgery should be considered only for patients with severe obesity who have not been able to lose weight with other treatment options and who are at high risk for developing other life-threatening health problems. The goal of these types of surgeries is to modify the gastrointestinal tract to reduce the amount of food that can be eaten.

Behavioral Therapy

A successful weight loss plan involves changing eating and physical activity habits to new patterns that will promote successful weight loss and weight control.

Behavioral therapy can include strategies such as keeping a food diary to help recognize eating habits; identifying high-risk situations (having high-calorie foods in the house) and then consciously avoiding them; and changing unrealistic beliefs related to a patient's body image. A support network such as family, friends or a support group, is beneficial as well.

How Is Body Fat Measured?

There are two ways in which body fat is measured: **waist circumference** and **body mass index (BMI)**. Waist circumference is a common measurement used to assess abdominal (stomach) fat. People with excess fat that is situated mostly around the abdomen are at risk for many of the serious conditions associated with obesity. A high-risk waistline is one that is 35 inches or greater in women and 40 inches or greater in men.

BMI is a measure of weight in relation to a person's height. For most people, BMI has a strong relationship to weight. To calculate your BMI use the following equations:

English Formula

$$BMI = \left(\frac{\text{weight in pounds}}{\text{(height in inches) x (height in inches)}} \right) \times 703$$

or

Metric Formula

$$BMI = \frac{\text{weight in kilograms}}{\text{(height in meters) x (height in meters)}}$$

Healthy weight: BMI from 18.5 to 25   **Overweight:** BMI from 25 to 30   **Obese:** BMI 30 or greater

For adults, BMI can also be found by using the table below. To use the BMI table, first find your weight at the bottom of the graph. Go straight up from that point until you reach the line that matches your height. Then look to see what weight group you fall in.

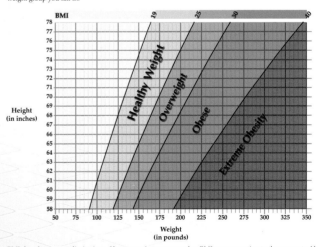

BMI does have some limitations. If a person is very muscular, BMI can overestimate the amount of body fat. It can also underestimate body fat if a person has lost muscle mass, as in the elderly. An actual diagnosis of obesity should be made by a health professional.

Obesity and Children

The prevalence of child obesity is increasing rapidly worldwide. In the U.S. alone, 1 out of 5 children is overweight. When compared to children with a healthy weight, overweight children are more likely to have an increased risk of heart disease, high blood pressure, and Type 2 diabetes. Children who are obese are also more likely to grow up to be obese adults. As with adults, lack of exercise, unhealthy eating habits, genetics and lifestyle all can influence a child's weight.

Doctors or healthcare professionals are the best people to help determine if your child is overweight. By considering your child's age and growth patterns, they can decide if the child's weight is healthy.

Health Risks Associated with Obesity

If you are obese, you have a greater risk of developing serious health problems. If you lose weight, the risk is reduced. The following is a list of diseases and disorders that can develop as a result of obesity.

A Brain
Psychological disorders (low-self esteem, depression), stroke

B Esophagus
Gastroesophageal reflux disease (GERD), heartburn

C Arteries
High blood pressure, arteriosclerosis (atherosclerosis, arteriolar sclerosis), high blood cholesterol

D Lungs
Asthma, sleep apnea (interrupted breathing while sleeping)

E Heart
Coronary heart disease, heart attack

F Gallbladder
Gallstones, cancer, inflammation of the gallbladder, gallbladder disease

G Pancreas
Insulin resistance, Type 2 diabetes, hyperinsulinemia

H Kidneys
Cancer, uric acid nephrolithiasis (stones in the kidneys)

I Colon
Cancer

J Bladder
Cancer, bladder control problems (stress incontinence)

K Bones
Gout (type of arthritis that deposits uric acid within the joints), osteoarthritis (degeneration of cartilage and bone in the joints)

Other possible health consequences of obesity include endometrial, breast, and prostate cancer; poor female reproductive health (menstrual irregularities, infertility, irregular ovulation, complications of pregnancy) and premature death.

Understanding Your Weight

83

Body Weight is Determined by Energy Balance

Obesity is excess body fat caused by long-term energy imbalance. Energy imbalance occurs when you consume more calories (energy intake through eating and drinking) than your body burns (energy expenditure through physical activity); this excess of energy intake is stored as fat in the body.

What Affects your Energy Intake? (calories consumed)

The amount of calories consumed and absorbed by the body.

What Affects your Energy Expenditure? (calories burned)

1. Metabolism – A process that produces the energy needed to run your body. The higher the metabolism, the more energy is burned.

Metabolism is affected by:

Muscle mass in the body – Muscle burns more calories than fat, even when the body is resting. A variety of factors can influence the amount of muscle mass one has, including:

- **Age** – As people get older, they tend to lose muscle mass.
- **Gender** – Men usually have more muscle mass than women.

Hormonal changes (menopause) – This can affect metabolism, but the effects are different for each person.

Genetics – The speed of metabolism can be inherited from your family.

Medications – Talk with your doctor about any prescription or over-the-counter drugs to find out more since some medications can increase or decrease metabolism.

Diet – Starvation, or abrupt calorie reduction, can cause significant drop in metabolism as the body tries to conserve energy to function.

Nicotine

Stress or emotional excitement

Body temperature due to fever or infection

Cold external temperature

2. Amount of physical activity – This includes any body movement throughout the day from walking through the grocery store, gardening, dancing, or any type of exercise.

3. Thermic effect of food – The energy required to digest, absorb, and metabolize food and drink.

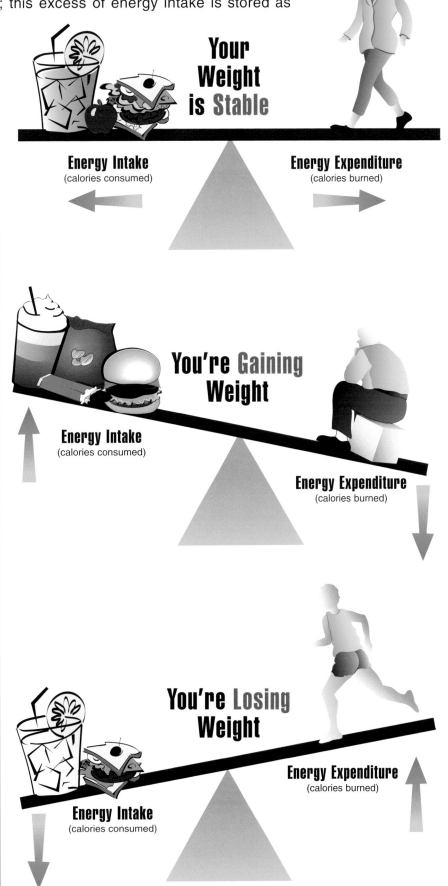

Your Weight is Stable

Energy Intake (calories consumed)

Energy Expenditure (calories burned)

You're Gaining Weight

Energy Intake (calories consumed)

Energy Expenditure (calories burned)

You're Losing Weight

Energy Intake (calories consumed)

Energy Expenditure (calories burned)

How to Lose Excess Weight

Set a reasonable goal for gradual weight loss – A realistic goal for weight loss is 5 – 10% of your initial body weight in 6 months; this translates to about 1-2 pounds of weight loss per week.

Improve your energy balance – Burn more calories through increased physical activity and metabolism than you consume through eating and drinking.

Focus on making small lifestyle changes – Over time these steps will add up to great results.

Track your diet and activity goals – Keep a diary or a log of all food intake and physical activity.

Talk to your doctor about other options – Medication or surgery, may be a choice if you have not achieved sufficient weight loss through diet and exercise.

Ways to Help Improve Your Diet

Reduce 500-1000 calories – Decrease energy intake and increase energy expenditure each day by making better choices of food and drink and increasing your physical activity. Thirty-five hundred calories is equal to one pound; if you can reduce 500 calories every day from your diet and with physical activity, you will lose 1 pound in a week!

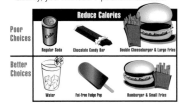

Recognize Your Eating Behaviors – One of the best ways to get a handle on eating behaviors is to keep a food dairy. Some common problems with eating patterns include:

- **Eating large portions**
- **Mindless eating and grazing**
- **Not eating enough fruits and vegetables**
- **Skipping meals**

Create a Supportive Environment

- **Request support** – Ask family members, friends, or co-workers to help/join you in your weight loss quest.
- **Replace unhealthy foods** – Keep healthy alternatives in your home and office.

Ways to Increase Your Physical Activity and Metabolism

Take the next step – Using the Physical Activity Pyramid, take the next step up (from where you are) to increase the number of calories burned. Talk to your doctor about any medical limitations.

Look for ways throughout the day to be more active – Go on a walk break or take the stairs. Break your activities into 10-minute blocks and try to add up to at least 30 minutes total per day. Track your activities every day with an activity log.

Add strength training – Use hand weights or resistance bands to increase muscle mass. This will increase metabolism and burn more calories.